Clear
Cane
Chronicles

CLEAR CANE CHRONICLES

Shaping the Future of Healthcare Through Person-Centered Care

Cynthia Overton, PhD

Published by Game Changer Publishing

Medical Disclaimer: The information contained in this book is provided for educational and informational purposes only and is not intended as medical advice, diagnosis, or treatment. It should not be used as a substitute for professional medical advice, care, or treatment from a qualified healthcare provider. Always seek the advice of your physician or other qualified health professional with any questions you may have regarding a medical condition or treatment. Never disregard professional medical advice or delay seeking it because of something you have read in this book. The author and publisher disclaim any liability, loss, or risk, personal or otherwise, that may be incurred as a consequence, directly or indirectly, of the use or application of any information presented herein. If you think you may be experiencing a medical emergency, call your doctor or emergency services immediately.

Paperback ISBN: 978-1-968250-99-7

Hardcover ISBN: 978-1-969372-00-1

Digital ISBN: 978-1-969372-01-8

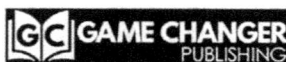

GC GAME CHANGER PUBLISHING
www.GameChangerPublishing.com

For Mom, Dad, Spencer, and Leslie—
who refused to accept "no" from anyone who couldn't say "yes."

LET'S STAY CONNECTED

Thank you for buying and reading *Clear Cane Chronicles*.
I'd love to stay in touch!

Please Scan the QR Code to Connect:

Clear Cane Chronicles

Cynthia Overton, PhD

FOREWORD

Welcome!

Before you dive into *Clear Cane Chronicles*, I want to offer a bit of context about what's ahead and talk about why person-centered care matters, how storytelling can open new perspectives on healthcare, and why patients, providers, and payers all have a role in advancing whole-person wellbeing.

The insights I share here are guided by experience and lessons gathered over a lifetime spent advocating for independent and community living by people with disabilities. My thoughts are anchored in the belief that the healthcare system should be person-centered and that it should work for everyone.

I write as someone who has spent a career championing access, dignity, and independence. In my work in developing the Americans with Disabilities Act and as convener of the National Advisory Board (NAB) on Improving Healthcare Services for Older Adults and People with Disabilities, I have seen how far we can go when lived experiences, real stories, and sound practices come together.

What stands out in this book is Cynthia Overton's personal story —a narrative that is both fun and engaging, full of candid moments that will take you on an emotional rollercoaster. You will laugh with her, feel the high stakes of her journey, and find plenty of space to pause for learning and reflection. This is not just another clinical textbook or self-help book; it is an experience—a journey richly told, where heartfelt scenes and humor are woven throughout. Cynthia's storytelling invites you to see healthcare differently, showing how warmth, honesty, and resilience can turn even the most challenging situations into impactful lessons.

Cynthia uses storytelling about her own experience to help readers understand formal frameworks that advance person-centered care and to illustrate, both emotionally and analytically, how these approaches can inform updates to policy and practice. She builds on this by connecting her experiences to findings from medical research and evidence-based practices, demonstrating the broader applicability of her insights.

As you read, you will discover how Cynthia uses her story to help patients and their families, payers, and providers understand formal frameworks like the NAB's Six Principles and the Picker Principles.

These frameworks matter because they help us treat patients as people first, with unique interests, preferences, and needs. Cynthia brings these principles to life throughout her book through her candid observations, notes of appreciation, honest reflections when the system misses the mark, and insight into how things can work better.

Cynthia offers a rare and detailed window into her experience transitioning into disability, and beautifully demonstrates through her story the need for inclusive infrastructure, supports, and services that allow everyone to thrive. Whether or not you have a disability, you will be certain to see how disability inclusion ends up improving daily life for everyone, by no means just for people with disabilities.

When you pick up this book, you will do more than just read. You will be equipped with conversation starters for patients, providers, and payers. Be prepared for meaningful discussions that will spark curiosity, expand your perspectives on healthcare, and uncover both barriers and assets that influence health outcomes.

I am so happy that you made the decision to pick up this book and immerse yourself in the world of person-centered care. May *Clear Cane Chronicles* serve as a source of knowledge, encouragement, and even laughter as you do your part toward building a comprehensive healthcare system that works for individuals in both clinical and community settings.

— Lex Frieden, Professor, Advocate, and Convener of the
National Advisory Board on Improving Healthcare Services
for Older Adults and People with Disabilities

July 2025

PREFACE

Chapman University administers an annual survey to understand what Americans fear most. Consistently, "a loved one becoming seriously ill" ranks near the top, coming in second in the most recent survey.[1] I can totally relate—not just as someone fearing for a loved one's health, but as the loved one who has been seriously ill.

In 1997, I had an arteriovenous malformation (AVM) removed from the C6-C7 region of my spinal cord. We'll get into that journey soon, but here's what I'll say for now: if a diagnosis is hard to pronounce, it usually isn't a good sign. For context, data from a 2009 study show that when I was diagnosed in 1997, only about 300 people in the U.S. were treated in hospitals for spinal AVMs or similar conditions each year—making it exceptionally rare.[2] In fact, you're about as likely to write a best-selling book as to be diagnosed with this condition. (And yes, I'm betting on a two-for-two here.)

As serious as my condition was, I know that many people face health challenges that are even more rare, unpredictable, or daunting. Whether you're navigating a crisis, trying to stay well, or you're somewhere in between, my message is the same: you deserve the best healthcare possible. And it starts with you. As the saying goes, "You have to love yourself first, before others can love you." The same is true for your health: empowerment opens the door to the care you need.

I wrote this book with a focus on patients, providers, and payers. Since we're all patients at some point, I'm devoting this preface to the patient in all of us. My hope is that you'll read it with your own health and experiences in mind, using its insights to take—or keep —an active role in your care. No sitting on the sidelines, letting healthcare just happen to you. We're in this together.

I can't close out this section without admitting that there have been times when fear kept me from facing my own health. But trust me, denial is not a good treatment option. The Chapman survey reminds us that fear, especially around illness, is universal. I think of taking care of your health like jumping into a cold pool—shock at first, but easier once you're in.

So, to all the patients—including the providers and payers among you—I'm excited to move forward together. Whether you're jumping right in or just dipping a toe, consider this your invitation to step in. Person-centered care is warmer than it looks.

— *Cynthia*

P.S. Since person-centered care is about the whole person, here's a little more about me: I love Korean dramas, *The Golden Girls*, and '80s music. I have a collection of clear canes—yes, there are favorites—and a firm belief that humor and humanity belong in healthcare, too.

ACKNOWLEDGMENTS

This book was made possible by the unwavering support of family, friends, and healthcare professionals who stood by me through one of the most challenging periods of my life. I am especially grateful to Mildred, Sterling, Spencer, and Leslie Overton; Fred Epstein, Renee Karibi-Whyte, Terence Thomas, Buzz Thomas, Linda Hotchkiss, Evelyn Simpkins, Alice Simpkins, Roberta Hinton, and Robbie Young, as well as my extended family, friends, healthcare providers, and coworkers who offered prayers, rides, meals, encouragement, care, compassion, and other support when I needed it most.

Writing this book was easier than living the story, but I could never have finished it alone. I owe heartfelt thanks to those who read drafts and provided invaluable feedback—Bushra Alawie, Ayanna Anderson, Carol Black, Harvey Goldberg, Linda Hotchkiss, Emily Jones, Jenny King, Joseph Olchefske, Mildred Overton, Dennis Pather, Tiffany Wood, and Jessie Wusthoff—as well as to

ACKNOWLEDGMENTS

the dedicated production and editing team who guided the manuscript to completion.

Many others planted seeds, offered strategic guidance, or provided encouragement throughout various points of my life, which gave me the confidence to turn this vision into reality. This group includes all of my manuscript reviewers, as well as Danny Allen, Michael Baran, Robert Birks, Cindy Cai, Eldred Ellis, Lex Frieden, Jessica Graham, Paolo Gaudiano, Esosa Imasuen, James Johnson, Catherine Leggett, Midori Noir, Spencer Overton, Sterling Overton, Phil Page, Brendan Pather, Tim Perry, Gary Rosen, Evelyn Simpkins, Tony Sparks, Orlando Taylor, Don Walter, Vince Wicker, and Jason Wright. I am also deeply grateful to my colleagues on the National Advisory Board (NAB). And to my 'Bu Crew friends— thank you for the laughter, support, and unwavering friendship that have made me smile, even during difficult times. (And yes, I know I'll get plenty of feedback at our next retreat.)

I'm deeply appreciative of the many people who took time to speak with me via Zoom or phone to offer their help along the way. These were patients, caregivers, physicians, health insurance professionals, healthcare administrators, marketing specialists, philanthropists, authors, and others. Each provided a unique perspective, and oftentimes, much-needed context and insights to fill important information gaps.

In addition to those who have advised me, I would like to thank all of the healthcare and disability advocates whose tireless efforts have paved the way for community living with dignity. My gratitude also extends to the Picker Institute and the National Advisory Board (NAB) on Improving Healthcare Services for Older Adults and People with Disabilities for their visionary leadership in creating principles that drive better health outcomes and support community living. I'd also like to thank Kathy Epstein for serving as a bridge to Dr. Fred Epstein's legacy, helping patients like me stay connected to his compassion and wisdom.

And finally, my deepest thanks to the individuals responsible for just about everything good in my life—my parents. My mother is fiercely loyal, endlessly opinionated, and always just a call away. She has always been in my corner, pushing me toward excellence whether I wanted it or not. My father's love runs deep, quietly showing itself through acts of care and steadfast support. He has always made me feel safe, and since childhood, made me the envy of many of my friends. My story would not exist without them.

CONTENTS

PART C: STRUTTING WITH SWAG

CHAPTER EIGHT

CHAPTER NINE

A NOTE ON PERSPECTIVE

TL;DR (Too Long; Didn't Read)

I wrote this "Note on Perspective" to help set expectations. But I have to admit that it's not the most exciting part of the book. Think of it like one of those pop-ups you get when installing software. Yes, it matters. No, it's not a page-turner. So if you skip this part, no hard feelings. I just ask that you keep these three things in mind:

- This book is written from a U.S. perspective.
- Everyone's experience is different, so I hope you'll explore other perspectives, too.
- I'm not a medical doctor, and this isn't medical or legal advice.

As you read, you might hit a few "what about…" moments. If you do, swing back here to see why I included some things and saved others. And if it's not in the book or this section—hey, maybe that's sequel material.

This Book Reflects My Healthcare Experience in the United States

This narrative explores *person-centered care* through the lens of my personal experiences receiving healthcare and navigating insurance in the U.S. While I hope readers from many backgrounds will find parts of my story relatable, I recognize that healthcare systems, resources, and cultural perspectives vary greatly around the world. Every country and community has its own unique strengths and challenges in delivering care. For readers outside the United States, this narrative offers a glimpse into the healthcare experience in this country.

This Book Addresses Policy, but Focuses on Person-Centered Care

Federal and local legislation, as well as non-legislative policies —including regulations, agency rules, administrative guidance, and internal procedures within healthcare systems—play a significant role in shaping how care is delivered, accessed, and experienced in the United States. These legal and policy factors are constantly evolving, so some details in this book may reflect practices that have since changed. Recognizing that policies, along with many other important influences, impact healthcare, I address policy issues to an extent, but the focus of my book remains person-centered care.

This Book Shares One Story from One Patient's Perspective

As I share my experience, I must acknowledge that my story does not represent every perspective. Every patient's experience is shaped by their unique background, identity, and circumstances, all of which can significantly influence the type of care they receive. Also, there are many sides to every story. Without the benefit of working as a medical professional or in the health insurance industry, I must emphasize the importance of seeking a variety of viewpoints to gain a broader perspective of how person-centered care can become standard in healthcare. With this in mind, I offer my book as just one data point among many. I encourage you to seek out and listen to the voices of other patients, as well as providers and payers, to gain a broader perspective on what person-centered care can mean in different contexts.

This Book Offers Insights on the Healthcare System—Not a Comprehensive Analysis

There is a lot to unpack in the healthcare system. While I touch on issues that have resonated with me, my focus remains on principles of person-centered care and how they've shaped my life. Reflecting on these decades after a significant health crisis offers a unique, long-term perspective. I've aimed to be thorough and to draw from publicly available resources as of 2025, though the body of information extends far beyond what's covered here. Through my story, I show how person-centered care, when practiced well or neglected, has shaped my health, well-being, and sense of agency. By sharing these experiences, I hope to illuminate practical opportunities for change, encourage others to consider their own roles, and show that better care is possible when we center the voices and needs of patients. My hope is that those conducting detailed analyses of healthcare systems will consider my perspective as one window into real-life impact.

This Book Does Not Offer Medical or Legal Advice

I am not a medical doctor. This book is informed by my personal journey as a patient and as someone who has navigated disability following a serious health event, as well as by my professional experience developing user-friendly patient education resources. The insights I share are rooted in formal frameworks that promote person-centered care, as well as in relevant healthcare research. Person-centered care is not a replacement for evidence-based medical practice or clinical expertise. In fact, evidence-based practice and clinical expertise are fundamental components of person-centered care. My purpose is to demonstrate how lived experience can inform and enrich the conversation about what comprehensive care looks like. Readers should consult qualified professionals for medical and legal advice regarding their care.

With Respect, This Book Does Not Cover Terminal Illness, Death, or Bereavement

Terminal illness, death, and bereavement are incredibly important topics that deserve the attention of those with specialized expertise and experience. If you seek guidance or assistance in these areas, I encourage you to consult individuals equipped to provide the help and attention you deserve.

This Book Uses Different Spellings

You may notice some spelling variations, such as *person-centered* vs. *person centred*. When referring to the Picker Institute, I use British spelling—*person centred*—to reflect their usage, which differs from U.S. publications that often use *patient-centered.*

This Book is a Reminder to Listen to All Patients (Not Just This Patient)

Finally, I want to reaffirm the importance of elevating the patient's perspective in healthcare. Patients have unique insights and lived experiences that are essential to advancing person-centered care. There is enormous potential for patients to become true partners—not just recipients—in the care process by working alongside clinicians, supporters, and community resources. I believe that embracing these partnerships can create a healthcare system that empowers everyone to lead fuller, healthier lives.

INTRODUCTION

HOW A CLEAR CANE BECAME MY SIDEKICK

I've carried a clear cane for half my life. It holds a story most people are too polite to ask about. I get it—asking what happened violates social etiquette—but I like sharing it because buried in that story are gems that can help patients speak up for better care, encourage providers to deliver more effective care, and position payers to support care that works for real people.

At twenty-six, my life revolved around friends, fun, and freedom. Overnight, I went from living my best life to lying in a hospital bed. Paralysis would soon follow, and my life as I knew it was thrown off course, all because of a spinal cord lesion I didn't even know existed.

This led to a crash course in hospitals, specialists, insurance appeals, and transitioning into a new life as a person with a disability—all without a roadmap. I was fortunate to receive high-quality medical care from a leading neurosurgeon, but looking back, what also shaped my recovery was something less obvious but just as powerful: providers who treated me like a whole person, not just a diagnosis.

Not everyone shares my experience. Across the U.S., a growing number of patients are expressing frustration and, in some cases, outrage about their experiences with the healthcare system. Stories of long waits, poor communication, insurance denials, and simply not feeling heard are all too common. Many patients are left fearful and uncertain about their health and angry at feeling disrespected, dismissed, or let down by the very system and people meant to help them.

These frustrations are no longer vented behind closed doors. They're broadcast online. Social media has become a megaphone for patients to share both their pain and their hope for something better. Online patient forums are filled with stories of unmet needs, emotional distress, and the search for dignity and partnership in care. In some cases, a single post or video can go viral, prompting public debate and, in some instances, serving as a catalyst for healthcare leaders to take steps toward improvement.

That's why the conversation is shifting. The answer isn't just better medicine; it's better care that responds to patients as people, not just cases.

PERSON–CENTERED CARE

That's what this book is about: person-centered care.

Person-centered care doesn't just make patients feel good. It addresses the whole person, including their goals, values, relationships, and environment.

Research indicates that person-centered care is associated with positive physical and social well-being, higher patient satisfaction, and more active engagement in care decisions.[1] It supports respectful partnerships between patients, families, and providers, helping ensure that care aligns with what matters most to each individual.[2,3]

Literature suggests that this approach also enhances provider satisfaction and care coordination and may reduce unnecessary interventions and costs by focusing on individualized needs and shared decision-making.[4] Ultimately, person-centered care can support better health outcomes, enhance quality of life, and foster a more responsive and sustainable healthcare system for everyone involved.[5]

Person-centered care should not be seen as merely an aspirational ideal. Patients, providers, and payers must work in alignment to make it part of everyday practice. This approach helps healthcare meet individual needs, improve outcomes, and transform lives.

Patient: An individual who receives healthcare services.

Provider: A licensed individual or organization that delivers healthcare services, such as doctors, nurses, therapists, hospitals, clinics, and health systems.

Payer: An entity that pays for healthcare services, such as health insurance companies, government programs like Medicare and Medicaid, and other third-party insurers.

I believe that a healthcare system can function at its best when patients are seen, heard, and respected; providers draw on the best science to deliver care in a way that meets each patient's unique needs; and payers earn the trust of members when their practices center members' health and well-being. Together, we all have the opportunity to make this a reality.

Traditional Clinical Care, Patient-Centered Care, and Person-Centered Care: What's the Difference?

My early experiences with healthcare followed the traditional model. Over time, though, there's been growing attention to "patient-centered" care and "person-centered care." These terms are often used interchangeably, but there are some important differences. Drawing on common descriptions in the healthcare literature, I've synthesized each to highlight how they differ.

Traditional clinical care is provider-driven: clinicians diagnose, treat, and expect patients to comply with their recommendations.

Patient-centered care moves the needle by respecting individual preferences and involving patients in decisions.

Person-centered care takes this further. It recognizes that a diagnosis is only one part of a person's life. It considers individual goals, relationships, environments, and beliefs. This approach addresses the whole person within the context of their life.

I like to think of person-centered care as healthcare for people who live in the real world, not in a medical chart.

Person-centered care empowers people to shape their care alongside providers, ensuring that treatments fit their real lives instead of letting a one-size-fits-all medical approach simply happen to them. In practice, this means honoring people's autonomy and unique experiences, and co-creating plans that reflect their values.

If you've seen television evolve over the years, you can probably spot the differences.

Traditional clinical care is like old-school network TV: one size fits all, take it or leave it.

Patient-centered care is cable: more choices but still bound by a system-driven schedule.

Person-centered care is the streaming era: personalized, on-demand, responsive. You log in, the system knows you, and it supports your choice in what to watch.

But not everyone has access to streaming-style healthcare. Some providers haven't been trained in person-centered care or may believe that they're already practicing it because they genuinely care about their patients. Some patients may not be aware of person-centered care, or may not feel empowered to speak up about their needs and preferences. Many payer systems aren't designed to support it. However, the call for change grows louder as more patients turn to social media to share their stories.

That's why I wrote this book: to show what person-centered care looks like when it works—and the downside when it doesn't. I hope patients find tools to advocate for themselves, that providers feel compelled to build on their clinical expertise by putting person-centered care into practice, and that payers recognize that investing in strategies that advance person-centered care leads to better health, greater satisfaction, and more sustainable, value-driven results.

FRAMEWORKS THAT ADVANCE PERSON-CENTERED CARE

I draw on two formal frameworks to describe my experiences and connect them to the concept of person-centered care. First, I use the Picker Institute's Eight Principles of Person Centred Care to reflect on my experiences within formal healthcare settings. Second, I reference the Six Principles to Modernize the Healthcare Infrastructure developed by the National Advisory Board (NAB) on Improving Healthcare Services for Older Adults and People with Disabilities to discuss healthcare as it relates to community living.

It's important to remember just how much progress has been made in the way we think about person-centered care. Person-centered care wasn't exactly trending in 1997 when I was hospitalized. Asking for person-centered care would've been like ordering an oat-milk latte and a gluten-free muffin in 1997: technically possible but definitely not on anyone's menu. Today, we have frameworks that serve as practical tools for advancing person-centered care. These tools help patients advocate for their care, providers deliver care that truly meets individual needs, and payers support care that actually works.

These types of frameworks represent the kind of care that is increasingly expected.

The Picker Institute's Eight Principles of Person Centred Care:[6]

- Fast access to reliable healthcare advice
- Effective treatment by trusted professionals
- Continuity of care and smooth transitions
- Involvement and support for family and carers
- Clear information, communication, and support for self-care
- Involvement in decisions and respect for preferences
- Emotional support, empathy, and respect
- Attention to physical and environmental needs

The Six Principles to Modernize the Healthcare Infrastructure developed by the National Advisory Board (NAB) on Improving Healthcare Services for Older Adults and People with Disabilities:[7]

- Improve health and well-being through individual empowerment and system coordination

- Achieve community inclusion and full participation
- Ensure full access to services and supports
- Value dignity and choice
- Achieve access to meaningful work and activities
- Accelerate access to innovative technologies

The NAB principles are especially important for older adults and people with disabilities seeking independence and long-term community inclusion, which are goals I share as I transitioned from hospital to home.

Safety is a fundamental and essential component of high-quality healthcare. Although the frameworks do not devote a standalone principle to safety, safety is inherently embedded throughout the core values of the principles. For example, Picker principles involving clear information, smooth transitions, and involvement in decisions can help prevent errors, reduce confusion, strengthen continuity, and provide an extra layer of protection for safer outcomes. NAB principles, such as ensuring full access to services and supports, can help detect issues early and enable effective contingency planning to maintain safe environments. These are just two examples of how the Picker and the NAB principles help patients, providers, and payers turn standard practices into safer practices.

In the chapters ahead, I'll revisit Picker and NAB principles through moments in my care: the good, the bad, the absurd, and the transformative. I don't come to this as a medical expert, but I am an expert at being a patient. If there's one thing I hope you take from this book, it's this: better care is possible when we all take action. Patients speak up, providers work together and partner with patients and payers, and payers support care that fits real lives.

I draw on the Picker and NAB principles as a shared approach for focusing on what matters most to people, rather than a prescription for every step. These frameworks support flexible thinking and collaborative problem-solving as needs, goals, and systems evolve. In some instances, the connection between my experience and these principles may not be obvious when viewed in isolation. However, those links become more evident when considered alongside the context provided with each principle, which is available in Appendix A at the end of this book.

HOW THE BOOK IS STRUCTURED

Part A, "Hospital Hopping," recounts my experience of being hospitalized and draws on the Picker Institute's principles to illustrate person-centered care in practice. Part B, "Elevator Dreams," explores my transition into life with a disability and uses the NAB principles to examine how person-centered care was present or absent throughout my healthcare and recovery. Part C, "Strutting with Swag," brings you into my life today, exploring both what it means to thrive while managing ongoing health challenges and the financial and policy forces that shape access to person-centered care in the United States.

Throughout the book, you'll find conversation starters for patients, providers, and payers as they consider their role in person-centered care. I close with practical thoughts on how each of us can help move healthcare forward—whether you're receiving care, delivering it, or shaping how it works. This is more than a memoir. It's a call to action for everyone concerned about healthcare. You'll have a front-row seat to what can happen when person-centered care works, and what's at stake when it doesn't. Whether you're a patient, a provider, or a payer, my hope is that you'll find practical ways to make healthcare more humane, more collaborative, and more effective.

"If you only had one car to last your entire life, you would take extraordinary care of it. Your body is the only one you'll ever have, so treat it just as well."
—Attributed to Warren Buffett

PART A: HOSPITAL HOPPING

THE (NOT SO) FINE PRINT ABOUT PART A

Part A, "Hospital Hopping," covers seven weeks across three hospitals and insurance appeals for spinal cord surgery coverage. I share what it's like having your life upended overnight, navigating tests, hospital routines, and red tape that makes tic-tac-toe feel like a Rubik's Cube. Despite these challenges, I consider my story a success.

Chapters 1-4 explore:

- Hospital admission, diagnosis, and adapting to hospital life
- Finding the right doctor and managing insurance
- Life-changing surgery and recovery in a new city
- Learning to walk again in rehabilitation

Throughout this section, I reflect on my experience through the lens of the Picker Institute's Eight Principles of Person Centred

Care—highlighting what supported healing and where the system fell short. Each chapter ends with conversation starters for patients, providers, and payers working to advance truly person-centered care.

ONE

FROM PARTY MODE TO PATIENT

THE DAY EVERYTHING CHANGED

"You need to go to the hospital now."

It took a minute to process the words coming out of my doctor's mouth. It was a Monday afternoon, and I was reporting back to her with yet another mystery symptom.

I'd started noticing changes a few months prior. Out of nowhere, I'd have moments of stillness when I knew what was happening around me, but my mind decided it wasn't going to let my body move. I went through periods where a few fingers on one hand would lock up, and I'd have to manually unlock them with my other hand.

Then there was the unbearable pain in the center of my upper back, which I attributed to a car accident. It surfaced mostly at night and sometimes throughout the day with each step that hit the floor.

I decided to get it checked out, but I had to do a bit of research since I didn't have a primary care physician at the time. This was before online reviews, so I ended up doing what we all did back in the '90s. I picked a doctor based on convenience. His office was a five-minute drive to my parents' house in Southfield, Michigan, a suburb of Detroit. Plus, nothing says "trust" like good parking.

I remember spending a considerable amount of time in the waiting room. Eventually, I was escorted to an exam room, where I waited some more. When I finally heard the doctor's name called from the hallway, I expected the door to open any moment. Nope. Turns out he had a call from his wife. This was before cell phones, and he was so loud that he sounded like he was on a phone right outside my door. They seemed to be discussing a real estate decision. At that point, I made a decision of my own: I got dressed and walked out.

I ended up picking another doctor but using a different approach, hoping for better luck. Instead of finding someone close to my parents' house, I found a doctor closer to my apartment in downtown Detroit. She ordered a stress test, which involved walking on a treadmill while connected to wires monitoring my heart activity. That test came back normal, so she had me wear a heart monitor for a few days. I had to carry a cross-body bag containing a small device with wires attached to my skin. That one looked fine, too. Since neither test found anything wrong, I must have been fine, right?

Well, not so fast. A few weeks later, my left leg just stopped working correctly, almost like it had fainted. It reminded me of someone who'd had way too much to drink and could only walk with one arm around a friend's shoulder. My leg was the lush, and the rest of my body was the friend carrying it along.

Earlier that day, a colleague had told me about someone who'd had a similar problem requiring leg surgery. At the time, I thought leg surgery was the worst-case scenario, and I hoped for a different prognosis. Clearly, I didn't understand human anatomy. What I'd face down the road would be much worse, and it has made me cautious about what I ask for.

"You need to go to the hospital now."

I had to replay her words in my mind for them to finally resonate, and then I did what any twenty-six-year-old would do: I proposed a counteroffer. "I have a hair appointment after I leave here, but Friday could work." After all, I was outside of the twenty-four-hour cancellation window and didn't want to pay that fee for a canceled hair appointment.

She paused and stared at me. Then she replied in a slightly lower tone while staring at me as if she were holding in a secret, "You don't understand. You have to go to the hospital now. We could be dealing with a stroke."

I called my mother from the doctor's office to let her know what was happening. I told her I could drive myself to the hospital, but she insisted on picking me up and taking me. She was expecting a group of women at her house for a meeting, but this was in 1997, way before group text chats, so she had to tape a note to the door explaining that the meeting was off.

While waiting for my mother, I wondered what being admitted to the hospital would be like. On TV, there's always a lot of commotion around hospital admissions. My memories were all of intense scenes, like accident victims arriving by ambulance and being rushed through the emergency room on a gurney, or a woman in labor lashing out at her husband in excruciating pain.

My experience was less dramatic. It was like checking into a hotel, just with more rules and no minibar. I could do without the minibar—after all, it was my drunk leg that had landed me in the hospital in the first place—but those rules, they hurt. One rule was especially painful: no outside medicine. I'd grown accustomed to taking two Tylenol each evening before bed. It helped control my back pain, which I thought had been caused by the car accident.

Since I was checking into the hospital with full insurance, the thought of bringing my own medicine never crossed my mind. I mean, who brings sand to the beach? I figured that asking for some Tylenol would be like ordering up some room service.

But when I tried, I heard, "I'm sorry, we can't administer any medication at this time. We need to find out what's going on with you first." The nurse on duty seemed nice, but in my mind, she must have been new and clearly didn't understand that a couple of Tylenol pills would be okay. I didn't need her anyway.

Even though my brother and I were grown, my mother still carried her "mom purse." That meant I had access to an arsenal of supplies: tissues, safety pins, Tylenol, you name it. So, when the nurse left, I casually pointed to my mom's purse and asked for the medicine.

By then, my father had arrived, and he was standing on the other side of my bed. She made eye contact with him and turned to me with the disappointing news: "The nurse said no."

I was confused. How could my mother take the nurse's side? If Yelp had been around back then, I would have pulled out my iPhone (which also hadn't been invented yet) and given that hospital a one-star review: "Worst healthcare ever. I've never experienced such horrible treatment in a hospital before in my life" (which, technically, would have been true since I had never stayed in a hospital before that). Okay, I wouldn't have done that. I just would have threatened to do it in my mind.

I looked at the clock, worried that the pain would begin at any moment. It always surfaced once my body had decompressed from the day. I started to beg. I was like Bruce Banner pleading with the bad guy not to make him angry so he wouldn't turn into the Hulk.

Then the pain began. It was excruciating.

I yelled, I cried, and I kept begging my mom for help. All I needed were two little pills, but she refused over and over again. As I think back on that time, so many years ago, I never considered what it was like for my parents, for them to watch their child in so much pain and accept the blame for not making it go away. We had conflicting priorities. I was concerned about my immediate interests. They were focused on my *best* interests.

I eventually dozed off, probably from wearing out my body with so much fussing, but the sleep didn't last. In the middle of the night, a mystery woman was transferred into the bed next to mine. I couldn't see her because the curtain separating our beds was closed, but I sure could hear her. After they dropped her off, she went on and on and on about the discomfort she was experiencing. By no means was she ranting. Instead, her grumblings were more like polite, "clear-your-throat" types of complaints, almost like she was "concerning" rather than "complaining."

Nurses responded by coming in and listening, but they didn't do anything that made her more comfortable. I don't know if the staff didn't believe her or if there was nothing they could do to help. I just know what I couldn't do, and that was sleep because of all the commotion.

Just as I started to doze off, the beeps from the machines on her side of the room started. The medical team came in, and a nurse escorted me out of the room and into the visitors' lounge. It was the middle of the night, so I was the only one there. The nurse brought me juice and a snack. Even though I wasn't really hungry, I ate it anyway—maybe as a way to distract myself from the guilt that I felt for complaining (not "concerning") in my head about all the noise the woman was making when she was just trying to get some relief.

I must have waited for twenty minutes before the nurse returned to escort me back to the room. When I walked in, the mystery woman was gone. I asked the nurse what had happened to her, but she wouldn't tell me. The bed remained empty throughout the rest of my stay.

The next week was dedicated to finding the actual problem in my body. Until then, I'd only focused on the symptoms: the locked fingers, the dragging leg, the unbearable back pain. Now, it's obvious, but back then, it didn't occur to me that addressing the actual problem, the root cause, might provide some relief from the symptoms.

Finding the problem involved a barrage of tests, which meant countless wheelchair rides around the hospital. But it wasn't until I underwent the mother of all tests, the MRI, that my problem was detected.

MRI stands for magnetic resonance imaging. It's a scan that creates detailed pictures of the soft tissues inside your body—like your brain, muscles, and organs—and it can detect abnormalities like tumors and injuries. If you're lucky, you're in and out in fifteen minutes, but I've read that they can last for up to an hour and a half.

I've had about ten MRIs in my lifetime. The first was the worst because it's such an odd experience. For starters, you have to be certain that you're not wearing any metals. Makes sense. The machine is like a giant magnet. I wore loungewear with no zippers but forgot the bobby pins in my hair. Rookie mistake. The pins scattered in the chamber, but thankfully, no harm done.

During an MRI, you lie down on what's like a conveyor belt, which slowly transports you into the machine. It's important to remain completely still so that the images are clear. No scratching, no sneezing, no nothing.

Someone described being in an MRI as like being in a coffin, but I disagree. Even though you don't need it, a coffin has more space to turn around. Plus, it has cushioning—also unnecessary, given the circumstances. Being in an MRI is more like being in one of those capsules they used to have at the bank drive-thru: it's hard and compact, and you get whisked in and out.

The MRI machine makes a loud jackhammer sound. During my first scan, instead of offering earplugs, the technician thought I'd be more comfortable with reggae music blasting inside the MRI chamber. But the music didn't drown out the construction noise. It just competed with it. The combination of reggae beats and relentless pounding was so absurd that I became fixated on the ridiculousness of the whole situation.

I will say that it was a distraction from the claustrophobia I had going into the chamber. Maybe that was the technician's intention. Who knows? I do know that I never showed up to an MRI again without a set of earplugs.

I was about five days into my hospital stay when I underwent the MRI scan. By that point, hospital life had become familiar: circling meal options on paper menus (remember, it was the '90s), random beeping sounds from machines, and patients in gowns tethered to IVs while they paced the halls, sometimes huddling outside for a cigarette.

Then there was the posse of doctors and nurses who flowed in and out of my hospital room. Some spoke extra loud, as if my nonexistent hearing aids were turned off. They'd make jottings in my medical chart that hung from the foot of my bed, out in the open for anyone to see. It was harder to get into my childhood diary than my medical chart back then. But that was hospital living, and it didn't take long for me to fall into the routine.

My mother also acclimated to the environment pretty quickly. She was there from the moment visiting hours started until the hour they ended. My father joined her in the evenings after work.

Even my brother and his wife flew into town, despite my explicit instructions to my parents not to tell anyone I was hospitalized. Admittedly, I was glad they came, but it was one more example of how, as a patient, your autonomy sometimes takes a backseat to the well-intended concerns of others.

I was lying in my hospital bed when I got the news.

A slender man in a white coat who appeared to be in his forties walked into my room. He was reading a document attached to a clipboard, and he struggled to make eye contact as he softly introduced himself as a neurosurgeon. I felt a sense of hesitance from him, which gave me the impression that he'd rather have been anywhere else in the world than in my hospital room.

"We need to discuss your MRI scans."

My mother reached for the notebook she'd been using to document conversations with the medical team. She was all about documentation: names, dates, times, and quotes. She was a regular Lois Lane. Not only did this help with managing my healthcare, but it sent the message, *I'm watching you, and I'm documenting everything that happens. I'll have the receipts if something goes wrong.*

Shortly after the surgeon began to speak, I stopped hearing complete sentences. It's almost like my mind was highlighting keywords and dismissing the rest. Lesion, spinal cord, rare, surgery, paralysis. Then the denial set in. "You can just talk to them about this," I blurted.

He paused for a moment and then said in a somber tone, "You need to hear this, too."

I figured that if he had to go through the anguish of delivering the news, the least I could do was be able to receive it. It took a minute, but eventually I came to understand that I had a lesion between the C6 and C7 region of my spinal cord. It had been present since birth and had grown throughout my lifetime.

I've always known that the spinal cord is linked to walking, but I'd never had a full appreciation of how important it is to your life. It controls your reflexes, how you perceive pain, how you regulate your body temperature, and your digestive system, not to mention your bladder and bowel functioning. Its reach is massive. Like, if Beyoncé were a body part, she'd be a spinal cord.

The lesion had hemorrhaged, which is why my leg wasn't working properly. The bleed caused nerve damage and led to "foot drop," making it hard to lift my foot when I walked. I was dealing with one of two things.

Option A: An arteriovenous malformation (AVM), which is essentially a bunch of tangled-up blood vessels trying to choke out my spinal cord. This was the good option.

Option B: A tumor and possible cancer.

There was no telling which one until the big reveal party on the operating table.

Now that the doctor knew we were dealing with a spinal cord lesion, he wanted to gather more information, so he ordered a spinal tap. I was told that I'd get a local anesthetic and would be awake during the procedure, but I still braced for pain since a needle to the back was involved.

It turned out to be a quick and easy procedure. In fact, I didn't really have time to panic. I felt something cold on my back, and before I knew it, I was done. My mother and brother waited in my hospital room for me to return.

Afterward, as I started to tell them all about it, I got distracted by a large bouquet of flowers on my nightstand. The sight of them caught me off guard, and I stopped mid-sentence.

"Where did those flowers come from?"

My mother glanced over at the flowers, looking just as confused as I felt. "Your coworkers sent them yesterday."

"Oh, okay."

I continued describing the spinal tap, but then I noticed a bouquet of flowers on the nightstand and changed the subject. "Where did those flowers come from?"

"The people from work sent them yesterday." My mother looked *really* confused as she answered this time.

"Oh."

I quickly pivoted back to my account of the spinal tap, explaining that it was so fast that they had actually finished the procedure when I thought they were just getting started.

But then I caught a glimpse of these flowers, sitting on the nightstand. "Where did those flowers come from?"

At this point, my brother and mother stared at each other. My brother thought I was joking around and laughed. My mother remained expressionless. She knew something was wrong.

I felt like my memory was slipping away from me like a bar of soap in the bathtub, and a sea of questions came flooding from my mouth. "Where did those flowers come from? How long have I been here? Why am I here? Where am I?" I felt like Laura Spencer in an old episode of *General Hospital*—minus the hair and makeup.

As quickly as my memory faded away, it came back to me.

But the most remarkable thing about the experience is that I remember it all. I actually remember having amnesia and then regaining my memory. I also remember feeling so desperate throughout the episode. When it was over, I had a greater appreciation for how difficult it must be to deal with challenges impacting brain functioning, *especially* when you're aware that your brain is not working the way you want it to.

Turns out there's a tiny, rare chance of experiencing temporary amnesia after a spinal tap. Not to complain, but a heads-up on that would've been helpful. Even if *I* forgot, my mother would've had it written down in her notebook.

But seriously, just because something is rare—like cognitive changes, or even my AVM—doesn't mean it can't happen. Sometimes, those fine-print possibilities become your big-time reality.

I have no idea about the details surrounding the spinal tap results, but I do know that we needed a surgeon who could remove the lesion from my spinal cord. We were faced with a serious decision and had only one card to play. We could bet on the neurosurgeon who had diagnosed me, a board-certified surgeon who had performed four operations annually comparable to the one I needed, or we could hold out for a specialist in hopes of a better payout. It was an easy decision to make.

• • •

PERSON-CENTERED CARE DISCUSSION

Getting Diagnosed

I want to pause for a moment to draw a few connections and a few departures between my experiences and select Picker Principles. But before we dive in, you may notice that an example can relate to more than one principle—*great observation!* For these exercises, I link each example to just one principle, but I encourage you to keep connecting the dots. If you'd like to review all eight principles and their explanations, they're listed at the end of the book in Appendix A.

Alignment With Person-Centered Care

Picker Principle: Fast Access to Reliable Healthcare Advice

When my leg finally gave out, my referring doctor didn't hesitate—she told me to go straight to the hospital. There was no waiting for a referral or "let's see how you feel in a week." Thanks to my insurance, I was admitted immediately and began undergoing the necessary tests.

In Picker-speak, this is fast access to reliable healthcare advice: seeing the right professionals and getting answers quickly, even if it means canceling a hair appointment. Unfortunately, research demonstrates that my experience isn't necessarily the norm. One study found that paperwork, bureaucratic procedures, and inadequate communication, among other administrative factors, can lead to delays in care.[1]

Quick and reliable care means that health concerns can be identified and treated before they escalate, reducing the risk of complications. And when you don't have to wait or fight for attention, you can focus on healing instead of navigating red tape.

Picker Principle: Involvement and Support for Family and Carers

My hospital room quickly became "Overton Central," with my family setting up what felt like a full-time command center. The medical team didn't just tolerate their presence—they welcomed it, answering my mom's endless questions and never flinching as she took notes on every conversation.

Helping us understand what was happening took time, but what we learned empowered us to make decisions moving forward. My experience aligns with perspectives that families provide context, care, and continuity that shape health and decision-making, serving as a foundation for health and well-being.[2]

Picker Principle: Involvement in Decisions and Respect for Preferences

Although the diagnosing doctor was polite, respectful, and professional—all hallmarks of good bedside manner—person-centered care goes beyond that. He was thorough with testing and went through multiple channels until he identified the problem. When explaining the test results, he pulled me back into the conversation when I was being dismissive and leaving my family to deal with the tough conversation.

Because the neurosurgeon involved me directly to ensure that I had all the information needed to determine my next steps, I was an active part of my care, even though the news was difficult. On top of this, research shows that engaging patients in their care is associated with better outcomes and satisfaction.[3]

Opportunities for Person-Centered Care

Picker Principle: Continuity of Care and Smooth Transitions

As positive as many aspects of my care were, transitions between teams within the same facility revealed a lack of communication that disrupted continuity. The team conducting my spinal tap clearly explained the procedure itself, but there was no handoff or shared plan between them and my primary care team. No one was designated to explain potential side effects—even the rare ones—and no one followed up afterward. As a result, my family and I had to face the disorienting effects of temporary amnesia alone. This gap wasn't just a missed conversation, it was a missed opportunity for a smooth, coordinated transition that would have honored the principle of continuity of care.

As a patient, I don't know if not disclosing potential side effects was a conscious decision because the risk was so small, or a regrettable oversight. I just know that TV commercials for prescription medications always list possible side effects—even if they're rattled off at lightning speed. At least they issue a warning.

I get that hospitals are busy places. But no matter how hectic things get, it's critical to consider what the patient is experiencing. Research shows that clear and empathetic communication, including preparing patients for possible side effects, is a core component of effective practice.[4] Ironically, in my case, the side effect that went unmentioned was confusion itself.

I don't want to complain too much, because the experience resulted in a story that has delighted crowds at cocktail parties for decades. Still, this not-so-smooth transition has left a lasting impression, and highlights where person-centered care in my experience fell short.

Picker Principle: Attention to Physical and Environmental Needs

The most chilling moment during my hospital stay wasn't about me. It was about the patient who briefly shared my room before disappearing into the night. She repeatedly expressed that she was in pain, but her distress was ignored. Turns out she's not alone. One poll conducted by HealthCentral, a website dedicated to chronic health found that 94% of its audience reported that their doctors had ignored or dismissed their symptoms.[5] While this was not a rigorous or representative study, the poll draws attention to patients' concerns about feeling overlooked.

Watching this distressing situation unfold made me appreciate the importance of listening to patients when their bodies are signaling that something is wrong. Research summarized in a review abstract indicates that dismissing patients' symptoms can lead to serious consequences, including healthcare avoidance, delayed diagnosis, and emotional harms such as shame, anxiety, trauma, and suicidal thoughts.[6] Just because an expert doesn't immediately understand a problem, doesn't mean it isn't real. Witnessing what happened to the patient who briefly shared my room underscored the importance of attentive, responsive care.

Picker Principle: Clear Information, Communication, and Support for Self-Care

Reflecting on my hospital experience, I realize how little emphasis was placed on empowering patients with helpful education resources about their prognosis and conditions. Providers shared diagnosis and answered questions, which was empowering. But this support was limited. There were no patient-friendly resources offered to help us understand care, rights, or what to expect.

Today, patients and families have far more options to access resources and understand their rights, to help with decision-making and care management. Entities including The Joint Commission,[7] CARF,[8] the Model Systems Knowledge Translation Center,[9] the National Library of Medicine,[10] and the National Institutes of Health (NIH)[11] are widely recognized for providing trustworthy and user-friendly health information for the general public.

Clear information equips patients to participate actively in their care, reducing anxiety and improving health outcomes. When patients and families are empowered with reliable resources and support for self-care, they are better prepared to handle challenges, advocate for themselves, and recover with greater confidence. Even as information becomes increasingly available, raising awareness and ensuring that patients know how to find and use these resources remain crucial.

• ● •

CONVERSATION STARTERS

I've developed a few questions to help patients, providers, and payers reflect on how person-centered care shows up or falls short in their experiences. There are no right or wrong answers here, just opportunities to spark conversations and explore what person-centered care looks like (or could look like) in your setting.

For Patients, Providers, and Payers

Reflecting on the narrative in this chapter, are there additional moments where Picker principles were exemplified or fell short?

For Patients

1. How have you noticed principles of person-centered care throughout your own healthcare journey?
2. When was a time you felt truly listened to by your care team? What made that experience different?
3. What resources or programs are available through your

healthcare providers to help patients and their families actively participate in care and decision-making?

4. How have you or your family been invited to share your values, goals, or preferences when making decisions about your care? How did that affect your experience?

For Providers

1. What framework guides your organization's approach to person-centered care? How do you operationalize this framework? If your organization does not operate under a framework, who would be best positioned to lead the process to identify one?

2. What specific resources or programs does your facility offer to help patients and their families actively participate in their care and decision-making? If they don't currently do this, who would be best positioned to take this on?

3. How do you "bring in" patients who appear detached or disinterested in taking an active role in understanding and managing their care?

4. Does your team do a good job of making sure that patients are aware of side effects that might occur from diagnostic procedures and treatment options?

For Payers

1. Based on recent patient satisfaction surveys or online reviews, how do your members rate their overall satisfaction with your services? How has feedback fluctuated over time?

2. What key themes have emerged from member feedback regarding what works well and what needs improvement when accessing care, communication, and other areas pertinent to person-centered care?

3. How do member experience ratings—such as those captured in CMS Star Ratings or similar quality measures—inform your quality improvement initiatives and strategic decisions?

4. How do you ensure individual member experiences are reflected and addressed, given that programs and solutions may be designed for groups or populations?

TWO

FINDING MY DREAM DOCTOR

AND GETTING INSURANCE TO SAY "I DO"

I was in the hospital for about a week before being discharged. Even though I was still able to walk, my parents insisted that I move back home. At the time, I was sharing a beautiful two-bedroom high-rise apartment in downtown Detroit with an old friend from high school.

We had a tight-knit group of friends in the building that we connected with for impromptu gatherings in each other's apartments or by the pool. Every day was like being on the set of *Living Single* or *Friends*, except that this was our actual life. But the spinal cord diagnosis flipped the script and sent me back to my childhood home.

I spent the first few days at home in my bedroom, grappling with the news and ruminating over the worst possible scenario. *I might have a cancerous tumor,* and *I might die.* I was so fixated on the possibility of death that I would go to bed wondering if I'd even wake up in the morning. I had access to care for the spinal cord lesion, but it never occurred to me or my family to seek psycholog-ical services or even explore mindfulness techniques to ease my anxiety. Everyone was just focused on getting this thing out of my spinal cord as soon as possible and as safely as possible.

I was so concerned about death that I even called my credit card company to close my account to make things easier for my family, *just in case*. When I told the customer service rep that I was getting my affairs in order, I could tell he was uncomfortable because he started fumbling over his words like he owed *me* money. It was the first and last time a credit card company tried to get me off the phone.

Figuring out the next course of action was my family's top priority. We understood the need to have this lesion removed from my spinal cord, along with the potential complications, particularly if the lesion turned out to be a malignant tumor. So, moving forward in the process on our own felt like a "Choose Your Own Adventure" exercise.

Admittedly, I didn't really know about exploring different options. My family, though, was a different story. They didn't have a lot of money, but they knew how to navigate systems. My father worked as a government administrator, so he was ready to deal with any bureaucratic hurdle that came his way. He'd mastered the art of cutting through red tape. My mother worked with students with special needs, evaluating, designing, and implementing interventions. With her background, she was ready to assess my needs, document every medical conversation, and anticipate challenges I might face both in and out of the hospital.

Then there were my brother and sister-in-law, along with a family friend, who had recently graduated from law school. They were prepared to explore all legal options to secure the care that we needed.

On top of this, I had a cousin who was a physician and another cousin who was in medical school. They served as our resident experts, clarifying medical jargon and explaining treatment options. Having medical insurance was not enough—I needed the backing of a powerhouse team to secure the best possible outcome.

Our top priority was finding a neurosurgeon who specialized in removing spinal cord lesions. The medical staff at the hospital was great in terms of running tests and explaining my problem, but they did not offer any viable leads for a specialist to conduct the operation. So, we circled back to the primary care physician who had ordered the initial tests and referred me to the hospital to see if she had any suggestions. Not only did she not have any recommendations, but she also refused to return any of our follow-up calls. She actually ghosted us. We suspected that she was concerned about medical liability, but we were laser-focused on finding a surgeon who could remove the lesion, so we kept things moving and continued the search.

Persistent phone calls and questions led us to the most experienced spinal cord surgeon in the state of Michigan. It turns out that this guy had never met a degree he didn't like. He had an MD, a JD, an MBA, and a PhD—and the confidence to match. But here's the catch. He only performed about ten of these surgeries a year. Now, I know that practice makes perfect, but not on me. He was nice, but I needed someone who specialized in my specific condition, rather than someone who worked across a variety of areas. So, the search continued.

We realized that we needed to broaden our search beyond the state, but that also meant that we were likely dealing with an out-of-network physician. Even if we found a surgeon willing to take the case, we still had to figure out how to pay for it. My brother and his friend were eager to put their law school training to use and started crafting arguments to persuade the insurance company to cover an out-of-network surgeon. They tackled this challenge head-on but also began working on a backup plan in case insurance fell through.

My parents looked into taking out a loan against the house, and even though my brother was buried in student debt from law school, he spotted a bank while getting a car wash and dropped in to see how much he could borrow. Whether through the insurance company or by getting a bank loan, my family was determined to get me the best care.

Finding a neurosurgeon out of state was no easy feat. Remember, it was 1997. Only about twenty percent of the U.S. population was online, and that was with a dial-up connection. Zero percent of the general population had a smartphone.

It felt like the Dark Ages when it came to accessing information. Believe me, if a Gen Z team had to compete in a reality show under these conditions, they'd be eliminated in the first round. But my sister-in-law had access to LexisNexis, a powerful research database containing detailed information on experts, including physicians. This led us to a neurosurgeon named Dr. Fred Epstein.

Dr. Epstein was based in New York City and was a pioneer in complex pediatric spinal cord surgeries. Each year, he performed hundreds of operations, including some of the rarest and most delicate spinal cord procedures, on patients from all over the world. No Cliff Notes for him—he basically wrote the book on rare spinal cord operations. The problem was that his contact information was not available on LexisNexis. It wouldn't be until years later that I learned that his home telephone number was listed in the public phone book so that anyone could get in touch with him.

It never occurred to us to reach out to someone in New York to check the phone book for us. Instead, one of my cousins, who's a physician, reached out to a friend from medical school who was based in New York to see if he knew Dr. Epstein. His response:

"Not only do I know him, I'm having breakfast with him in the morning. I'll tell him about your cousin."

Dr. Epstein sent word to my family to contact him. My father called him as soon as he received the news. The doctor's receptionist answered the phone and, after my father identified himself, said, "He's been expecting your call."

They discussed my situation, and Dr. Epstein instructed him to make copies of my MRI films and send them to him overnight by express mail. With help from my father's colleague, we found a service that could duplicate the films and sent them out right away.

Dr. Epstein reviewed the films and called my father, telling him that he needed to do the surgery and they needed to get me to New York as soon as possible because the lesion was at risk of hemorrhaging again. We still had no luck persuading the insurance company to pay for the surgery, but Dr. Epstein said if they changed their position, he'd accept whatever surgeon's fee they offered. The hospital fee was an administrative issue and out of his control.

Now that we had an expert to perform the surgery, we could focus on paying for it. After getting a formal "no" from the insurance company, my family reached out to everyone they knew who was remotely associated with the insurance company—employees, executives, and even politicians. In a final act of desperation, my mother went to see her friend, in her office at the same insurance company where I had coverage, to ask for advice. Her friend told her there was no way that they would pay.

My parents realized that they would need to take out a loan against their home to get the quality of care needed for the best possible outcome, even though I had health insurance. On the very morning that my mother was headed to the bank to complete the paperwork, the insurance company called. They agreed to cover the cost of the surgery.

• • •

PERSON-CENTERED CARE DISCUSSION

Navigating Specialists and Insurance

We've just covered a whirlwind of medical decisions, insurance negotiations, and specialist referrals. How did person-centered care shine through, and where was it absent?

Alignment With Person-Centered Care

Picker Principle: Effective Treatment by Trusted Professionals

Accessing effective treatment from a trusted professional was a pivotal part of my care, but it didn't happen by chance. Securing a surgeon with the right expertise took significant advocacy from my family. In the late 1990s, finding a specialist for my rare spinal cord procedure was challenging, and navigating insurance barriers added another layer of complexity. My family's persistence paid off, and I had access to a provider who offered the possibility of better health outcomes, greater peace of mind, and a genuine sense of partnership in care.

But despite today's apps and websites that offer contact information, professional histories, and reviews for providers, accessing effective treatment by trusted professionals can still be tough, especially for people with lower levels of health literacy, which is often associated with lower educational attainment. Studies demonstrate a correlation between education and better health outcomes, due, in part, to increased health literacy, exposure to advocacy training, and greater confidence navigating healthcare systems.[1]

As grateful as I am for the family into which I was born, this strikes me as incredibly unfair. This is just one example of how social drivers like education, advocacy, and support networks can shape access to healthcare. Until such disparities are addressed, stories like mine will remain the exception rather than the norm. Upholding the Picker Principle means that excellent care is available to all, regardless of one's ability to navigate complex systems.

Picker Principle: Involvement and Support for Family and Carers

Once my family connected with Dr. Epstein, he made himself available to our family and guided us through every logistical step. This involved answering all of our questions promptly, helping us navigate payment and insurance hurdles, and explaining how to obtain my MRI films for review. Taking just a few minutes to walk us through these details saved my family hours of confusion and frustration.

Research suggests that Dr. Epstein's approach is ideal, as engaging a patient's support system improves communication, reduces logistical stress and burnout, and empowers providers to take a more holistic approach to care.[2]

This kind of involvement and support for family and carers is at the heart of person-centered care. When healthcare teams treat families as true partners, they not only lighten their own workload but also empower families to advocate effectively, make informed decisions, and reduce stress during an already overwhelming time.

Picker Principle: Involvement in Decisions and Respect for Preferences

Although my family had to persist with the insurance company, we ultimately saw this principle in action when they agreed to cover my out-of-network spinal cord surgery. Choosing a neurosurgeon without deep expertise in my condition would have meant a higher risk of paralysis, incomplete removal, and even death. Our clear preference was to have an expert perform the surgery, and Dr. Epstein's experience gave me the best possible chance for an optimal recovery.

The risk of claim denial remains very much present today. An analysis of ACA marketplace plans found that 19% of in-network and 37% of out-of-network claims were denied in 2023.[3] Fewer than 1% of these denials were appealed, and when they were, about 44% were overturned on internal review, with the insurer ultimately paying the claim. A separate national analysis found that across all payers, roughly 70% of initially denied claims were eventually paid, typically after multiple rounds of review—a process described as costly and time-consuming.[4]

Data show that only 6% of denials are for lack of medical necessity, whereas about 18% are due to administrative errors—such as incorrect billing codes, outdated provider addresses, or even misspelled patient names.[5] All of this demonstrates that involvement in decisions and respect for preferences extend well beyond the exam room. In many cases, they require persistent, informed engagement with insurance systems as well.

Opportunities for Person-Centered Care

Picker Principle: Continuity of Care and Smooth Transitions

The involvement of my primary care physician ended abruptly when she stopped returning our calls and removed herself from my case. This sudden disengagement disrupted the continuity of care and made an already stressful situation worse. I recently learned that I likely experienced "patient abandonment," which is a breach of duty.[6]

At the time, there was little recourse—no widely used online reviews, complaint systems, or clear channels to hold providers accountable. Today, there are far more outlets to support account-ability in healthcare. Survey data from RepuGen, a platform used by providers to manage their online reputation, indicate that a majority of patients consider online reviews when selecting a healthcare provider, and that providers who respond thoughtfully to feedback can significantly improve patient satisfaction and trust.[7]

In addition, many insurers and health systems have adopted value-based payment models and pay-for-performance programs, which reward providers for delivering high-quality, coordinated care and maintaining patient engagement.[8] These models reward providers for meeting standards in communication, follow-up, and patient outcomes, reducing the likelihood of patients being left without support during critical transitions.

Research suggests that continuity of care is strengthened through early discharge planning, active patient involvement, and clear communication throughout the care journey.[9] Electronic health records, transition coordinators, standardized handoff protocols, and other tools help ensure that information flows smoothly between settings. This reduces the risk of patients feeling abandoned or lost in the system. When transitions are well-managed, patients and families can focus on recovery, rather than scrambling to fill gaps in care.

Picker Principle: Emotional Support, Empathy, and Respect

While most of my experiences with healthcare providers were positive, the emotional side of care was often overlooked. My doctors generally empathized with me and wanted what was best for me, but the focus was almost entirely on my physical health. Being told I could face death or paralysis was overwhelming, yet I was left to process those fears and emotions on my own.

Concerns like stigma, bias, and systemic barriers are often cited as roadblocks to mental health care in Black communities. But in my case, the mental health component just got triaged out. We had a finite amount of time, we were facing life or death, and in reality, we were accustomed to pushing through incredibly difficult social circumstances as part of day-to-day life. I share this not to excuse the gap, but to explain how easily emotional needs can be sidelined in crisis.

Looking back, I realize how much I would have benefited from someone who could have helped me work through the emotional impact of my diagnosis and treatment. Technical skill and medical expertise for my physical needs were critical, but person-centered care also means recognizing and addressing the emotional needs that come with a life-changing diagnosis. This would have probably eased anxiety, increased my confidence, and offered me more peace.

Picker Principle: Fast Access to Reliable Healthcare Advice

We eventually gained access to reliable healthcare advice (thanks to Dr. Epstein), but getting there felt like a reality show challenge. If our medical team had even just pointed us toward the right resources or specialists, our journey could have been far more efficient. But the reality is that providers are human, and it's impossible for everyone to know about every condition.

Moreover, the flow of information was far more limited in 1997 than it is today, which made it more challenging for both healthcare providers and patients to identify specialists.

A lot has changed since I had spinal cord surgery. Today, families seeking advice for rare conditions can leverage technology to find specialists and treatment centers with online databases, expert networks, and advocacy organizations.[10] Faster access to reliable healthcare advice—whether locally, across the country, or around the world—can lead to faster treatment and increase possibilities for better health outcomes.

• • •

CONVERSATION STARTERS

Patients, providers, and payers all face the administrative challenges that come with navigating health insurance. But there's no need to go through this alone. Here are some conversation starters to help spark productive discussions.

For Patients, Providers, and Payers

Reflecting on the narrative in this chapter, are there additional moments where Picker principles were exemplified or fell short?

For Patients

1. How do you find out what your insurance company requires when seeking a treatment, test, or specialist visit? Who is your first point of contact, and how do you make use of the expertise available from customer service, your doctor's office, an insurance case manager, or a patient advocate?

2. If you ever need to see a specialist who's out-of-network because they have unique expertise, what kind of paperwork or documentation will your insurance company want? Is there someone, maybe a case manager or patient advocate, who can guide you through that?

3. If your insurance denies coverage for a treatment or specialist, what immediate steps should you take to begin the appeals process? Who can help you with the required paperwork, and how quickly does each part of the process need to be completed to avoid missing important deadlines?

4. Does your insurance plan offer any case management or support services for people dealing with complex health issues? If so, how do you connect with those services, and what kind of help should you expect?

For Providers

1. When complex or out-of-network care is needed and coverage rules vary so much across insurance plans, how do you help patients and families figure out what is and isn't covered? What strategies or resources do you offer to guide them—even when you may not have all the answers?

2. When you believe out-of-network care is genuinely in a patient's best interest, how do you go about advocating for coverage with insurance companies? What have been your challenges and secrets to a successful approval? What could make the process more efficient or less burdensome for both providers and patients?

3. Are you aware of, and do you routinely inform patients about, case management or patient advocacy services offered by insurance plans that could help them navigate approvals and appeals?

4. How does your practice support patients and families through the insurance appeals process when coverage for necessary care is denied? What steps do you take to ensure your staff are trained to submit the required documentation correctly and quickly? What practices or tools have you found most helpful in avoiding delays and making the appeals process as efficient as possible for patients?

For Payers

1. How can you help members better understand their coverage details and what they'll be responsible for financially?

2. How do you support providers when they're working with your company on claim approvals? How do you minimize the time they spend on administrative tasks related to these claims so they can focus more on patient care?

3. How do you ensure that benefit information—whether in pamphlets, books, or online resources—is clear and accessible enough for members to understand what's covered, especially when care is complex or urgent?

4. Have you found that denying coverage for certain treatments or specialist care now can contribute to higher costs or diminished outcomes for both your company and your members in the future? How does your organization weigh these downstream risks when making coverage decisions?

THREE

SURGERY AND THE CITY

FROM HIGH HEELS TO HOSPITAL SOCKS

My family was off to New York City for the surgery. We had a family friend who had recently moved to New Jersey—close enough for a reasonable hospital commute—and she generously offered to vacate her apartment and move in with her parents during my hospital stay. With housing covered, the only major expenses my family encountered were airline tickets and a car rental, which they used to drive into the city every day to visit me in the hospital.

At this point, I had been on steroids to help manage the lesion in my spinal cord. What I didn't realize was that they were causing severe constipation. I was miserable. It felt like my belly was one big beach ball, just expanding more and more. I was so desperate, I spoke with anyone, and I mean *anyone*, who would listen to me talk about my bowels and my mission for relief. The pharmacist at a local drugstore recommended an over-the-counter gas medication—something pretty mild. I think my belly stopped expanding just long enough to chuckle at the tablets and then kept right on growing.

Once we arrived in New York, there was no time for sightseeing or even settling in. The very next day, my parents, brother, sister-in-law, and I were off to the city to meet Dr. Epstein. He'd requested a meeting with the entire family.

As we approached his office, we noticed that the nameplate next to his door just said "Fred." No "Dr." and no "MD." Just "Fred." We're talking about a world-renowned neurosurgeon, who goes by "Fred"—like the guy who fixes your car, Fred. I mean, even Mr. Rogers didn't go by just Fred. It was a little confusing.

He greeted us with a very warm smile as though we were old friends reuniting. One of the questions my mother asked was how to pronounce his name. "Is it Ep*steen* (rhymes with team) or Ep*stine* (rhymes with spine)?" He responded with a shrug, "It doesn't matter."

Dr. Epstein expressed an interest in all of us. When my mother told him that she was a teacher consultant and worked with kids with learning disabilities, he said, "Oh, I think I had a learning disability." This caught us all off guard. I mean, after all, this was the guy who was about to take a shovel to my spinal cord. My family tried to communicate with each other through our eyes, but Dr. Epstein quickly caught on. "Oh, don't worry," he said. "I'm fine. Everything is fine."

I found comfort in his reassurance, and now that I look back on things, I realize that calling himself just "Fred," not being concerned about how his name was pronounced, and finding common ground between himself and my mother's profession were his way of making meaningful connections with us. This was a person who pioneered groundbreaking surgical techniques for spinal cord conditions that had previously been inoperable, and he was focused on making us as comfortable as possible. Mission accomplished. He got to know us. He explained the procedure and what we could expect, and by the time our meeting was over, we all felt confident that we'd made the right decision.

On the day of the surgery, only one family member was allowed to accompany me in the area where I was prepped for the operation. That was my mother. Before going back into that area, I gave a letter to each of my family members—my mother, my father, my brother, and my sister-in-law—to express my love and gratitude, just in case things didn't work out as we'd hoped. I'd also written a letter to myself. After all, nobody warned me about the temporary amnesia after the spinal tap—and that was just a little tap. Now it was showtime, so there was no telling what would happen once they really started digging in. I wanted to be ready, just in case this turned into long-term amnesia. In the letter, I included where I was and why I was there. I also included information about each of my family members, with strict instructions to only leave New York with them.

The last thing I remember before being wheeled into the operating room was a conversation with the anesthesiologist. I told him about a friend who'd woken up during eye surgery, so I needed him to give me enough juice to keep me under, but not so much that I'd get amnesia (even though I was ready with my letters). He seemed amused that I was trying to help him do his job and assured me that everything would be okay.

The next thing I knew, I was awake in the intensive care unit. I couldn't feel my legs, but I was alive. Dr. Epstein did a test where he scraped the bottom of my feet to see what I could feel. Then he tried to get me to press up and down against his hand. Even though I was completely paralyzed, one leg felt stronger than the other, and I had a little sensation in the weaker leg. It felt like my wires were crossed—nothing with my legs felt intuitive. I actually thought that the doctors would think that I wasn't telling the truth because it just seemed ridiculous. But I had to tell Dr. Epstein what was really going on. His response: "That's how it's supposed to be." He also told me that the recovery process would get harder before it got better, but that the surgery had gone well. The lesion turned out to be an AVM. No tumor. No cancer. No going to sleep and not waking up.

My family stayed with me in the ICU until visiting hours ended. The ICU is an interesting place. My experience was so peaceful, and it almost felt like staying on the concierge floor of a hotel. I quickly learned that the ICU doesn't necessarily reflect the realities of the hospital experience. The next day, I was moved to the step-down unit, and the name says it all. It was a "step down" from the white-glove service I got in the ICU. Okay, maybe I'm not being fair, but that's how it felt.

The step-down unit is actually where patients go when they no longer need the constant monitoring offered in the ICU but still require more care than what's available on a typical hospital floor. It was full of noise and people, and reminded me of a scene from the old television show *M*A*S*H*, with everyone crowded together on little cots (although we did have proper hospital beds). Some might say I complained, but I was really just commenting, loudly and often, on the noise. In fact, I made so many comments that my care team waived the requirement for me to stay the full twenty-four hours and moved me to the room where I'd spend the next two weeks. Or more simply put, I got kicked out of step-down.

My new room had an amazing view of Manhattan. There was no way that I could have afforded that view at a New York City hotel. Here I was in the city that never sleeps, but sleeping would be my go-to activity for the next two weeks.

I shared the room with a woman in her 60s. She was a nurse who smiled a lot and was also there for spinal cord surgery. She had an adult daughter, but didn't tell her about the surgery so she wouldn't worry. Instead, she'd left a note on the kitchen table, just in case she didn't make it back home. Even though she was alone, her nursing background gave her the insight and confidence to understand what was happening and manage her care. The way she engaged with the staff made me think she might hop out of bed and pick up an extra shift.

Every day, my parents made the commute from New Jersey to visit me. They were very conscientious about bringing snacks for the staff because they wanted a way to draw them into my room to check on me. They also kept my room filled with cards and other small items that sent the message, "I've got people here who have my back." But really, every last person at that facility was so amazing that they would have checked in on me anyway.

Dr. Epstein visited my hospital room regularly to monitor my recovery, and always brought a sense of calm and reassurance. During one of his rounds, he even invited me to join him for dinner if I ever found myself back in New York. At the time, I wasn't fully aware of the impact Dr. Epstein had on me, but my mother later told me that my face would light up whenever he entered the room. Dr. Epstein had a remarkable presence—genuine, compassionate, and deeply committed to his patients. He was someone who truly knew his purpose in life and spent every moment pursuing it.

During my stay, the television program *20/20* was taping a segment featuring Dr. Epstein. I was doing my physical therapy in bed, and my therapist told me all about the taping. She made me wish I were out in the main part of the hospital, where all the action was. Turns out, Dr. Epstein performed spinal cord surgery on a dog named Tucket. But that wasn't the angle. The dog's family could not stand the thought of him being put down because of the condition and had sought out Dr. Epstein, who had agreed to perform the surgery if the family paid for the surgery of a child. And that's what they did.

My recovery process was really hard. The first thing I had to do was make a mental shift. My legs went from feeling like two strong baseball bats to two giant hot dogs. I had to adjust my thinking about the most basic things, like realizing I couldn't just get out of bed whenever I wanted. I couldn't just get up and go to the bathroom or take a shower.

The disruption in communication between my brain and my body didn't just affect my walking. I'd wake up in the middle of the night, knowing it was for a reason but not remembering why. I'd pee myself—yes, right there in the bed—and then it would hit me: "Oh, that's why I woke up. I had to go to the bathroom."

That was a very humbling experience, but it wasn't humiliating. I was dependent on others for help; I just couldn't do everything by myself. But any ounce of embarrassment I felt dwindled away after my first few encounters with the nursing assistants, who made me feel comfortable. These are the people who gave me sponge baths in bed (and no, it was not something to look forward to, like in the movies), put me on the bedpan, and helped me change gowns. Think of the most personal activities of daily living—they are the ones who helped me with them.

And here's the thing: gender was not a factor when it came to who was assigned to help you. You could be placed on a bedpan by someone you might be trying to flirt with at Starbucks if the circumstances were different. You did have the option to request a man or a woman to help, but there was a catch—if you exercised that option, it might take a bit longer to get help based on availability.

The hospital staff did their absolute best to respect patient preferences, but once I realized the potential for delays, I quickly removed gender from the equation and went with whoever was available. And you know what? There really was no difference in how I felt. The gender of the nursing assistant available to help with personal tasks had nothing to do with their quality of care. For me, it was all about their professionalism and the respect they demonstrated, which was always top-notch. Keep in mind that I didn't have modesty restrictions based on personal values or faith. What was optional for me might be non-negotiable for others.

Being in that position made me realize that my nursing assistants were some of the most underrecognized and critically important people I encountered during my entire stay in three different hospitals. They approach their jobs with professionalism and compassion, and I appreciate them so much. I wish every patient could have this experience—it makes being in the hospital so much better.

My nurses in that facility were also great. They always seemed genuinely happy to see me whenever they came in, though I'll admit, I was probably a lot easier to be around once I stopped "commenting" on all the noise.

As a spinal cord patient, I had to go through intermittent catheterizations to make sure my bladder was emptied. This meant having a tube inserted through my urethra into my bladder to drain the urine. I didn't really understand why it was necessary; I just knew it was uncomfortable.

So, when one nurse asked me if I wanted catheterization instead of simply stating that it would be done, I jumped at the chance and replied with a polite "no, thank you." I didn't realize how important it was—or that the nurse was keeping track. The nurse on the next shift noticed in my chart that I had "refused" catheterization. This, I guess, was technically true, but in my mind, it was just a simple "no, thank you," like turning down a wedding invitation from your ex. I probably would have chosen differently had I known it would go on my permanent record.

I continued with in-bed physical therapy at that hospital for the next two weeks. During that time, my family visited me every day. I was so used to their constant presence that the day they didn't show up until visiting hours were almost over is still burned into my memory. They needed a break, which, looking back, I completely understand. But at the time, it felt almost like a betrayal, or at least grounds to question their commitment (I know, that sounds ridiculous now). They'd spent the day sightseeing and ended up at the legendary Junior's for a meal and some cheesecake.

What I didn't realize then is that caregiver burnout is real. As a patient, it's hard to see that. At that stage of my recovery, I couldn't imagine the world revolving around anyone but me. Plus, nobody was speaking up to say, "Hey, I'm starting to feel stressed out. You're stable, so I'm gonna take a minute." Now I can see that their break gave them the space and energy to refuel and refocus on me, but at the time, I just felt kind of forgotten about.

As a caregiver, it can be hard to accept the reality of what's happening. Early in my hospital stay, my mother was so worried that I wasn't getting out of bed that she actually tried to lift me out herself. Intellectually, she knew I was receiving the best care possible, but emotionally, she just couldn't accept that my legs didn't work. She felt like she had to do something to speed up the recovery process and ended up trying to get me out of bed. That did not go well. I fell to the floor, and I felt terrible for her because that was the moment she truly realized that I was actually paralyzed.

The staff rushed in to help me back into bed. They were clearly alarmed—even though they kept their voices calm, I could see the shock on their faces. My mom was crushed, not just by what had happened, but by the reality that I had no use of my legs. Despite all the mountains she'd moved and the sacrifices she'd made (and was willing to make) to ensure that I received the best possible care, she still carries the guilt of that day, even years later.

Thanksgiving fell about ten days into our hospital stay. The staff was kind enough to allow my mother to bring in dinner so we could all have a sit-down meal together. We were used to large Thanksgiving dinners of fifty or more with extended family, but a dinner for five in a hospital room would have to suffice that year. My mother laid out a spread in the small visitors' room, which we ended up having to ourselves.

The dinner was much more ceremonial for me than a good time because I was in so much pain from the muscle spasms in my shoulder that developed after my surgery. I felt like I was being stabbed with an ice pick, and the only thing that remotely helped was an IV bag filled with ice, draped over my shoulder. I remember being rolled into the visitors' room in a wheelchair, having a plate, fake smiling for a picture with a disposable camera, and being rolled back to my bed. My family tried to be upbeat, but it was hard seeing me suffer. Still, it provided a sense of normalcy for me, which I appreciated. The circumstances were different, but our tradition of having Thanksgiving dinner as a family, albeit abbreviated, remained intact.

I was discharged from the hospital about two weeks after surgery, with plans to go directly to an inpatient rehabilitation facility in Detroit. Because my spinal cord injury made it difficult for me to control my bladder, I needed a way to manage urine during the plane ride home. When I asked a nurse how to handle this, she explained that my options were either to wear an adult diaper or to use a catheter.

At first, I was set on the diaper, but since my roommate was a nurse, I asked her what she would do. She said she'd definitely choose the catheter. I decided to go with her recommendation, and it turned out to be just fine. The only awkward part was when the security agent at the airport discovered my urine bag as she patted me down. She didn't even blink, though, which made the whole experience easier.

Once we landed, airport employees helped me transfer from a standard wheelchair to a narrow one that fit down the airplane aisle. The pilot himself rolled me from the plane to the curb, which was an unexpected and pleasant surprise. Then it was off to my third facility for intensive physical and occupational therapy.

• • •

PERSON-CENTERED CARE DISCUSSION

Confronting Surgery and Recovery

Chapter 3 covers some pretty personal details that put principles of person-centered care to the test. Here's how my experience aligned with and deviated from those principles.

Alignment With Person-Centered Care

Picker Principle: Effective Treatment by Trusted Professionals

Dr. Epstein's leadership and person-centered approach set the tone for exceptional care. As a pioneer in spinal cord conditions, he took time to understand my family and me, explained every step thoroughly, and showed genuine compassion before, during, and after surgery. Dr. Epstein's legacy continues as a model of how technical expertise and profound compassion can go hand in hand.

I believe that most providers are deeply committed to the well-being of their patients and want to demonstrate the level of care that Dr. Epstein provided to his patients. Yet many face intense pressure caused by staffing shortages, administrative burdens, extensive paperwork, and systemic inefficiencies.

What we observe as patients doesn't provide the full picture behind the scenes. Hospital leadership plays a crucial role in creating environments where care teams have the support needed to deliver person-centered care.

Research demonstrates that when providers and healthcare administrators effectively collaborate within a positive organizational culture that has inclusive leadership support and shared goals, care teams are better positioned to learn from mistakes, experience less burnout, and achieve improved patient outcomes.[1] In other words, when healthcare leadership creates the right conditions, providers can focus more on caring for the whole patient and less on navigating structural barriers.

Picker Principle: Emotional Support, Empathy, and Respect

The nursing assistants approached every aspect of my care with compassion, respect, and professionalism, always preserving my dignity, even during the most personal moments. Their presence made a difficult time feel less isolating and more manageable. This isn't every patient's experience, and I hope hospitals recognize the vital importance of these roles.

A grounded theory study shows that nursing assistants and other frontline caregivers play a significant role in shaping the patient experience, as their daily support and positive connections help patients adapt to hospital life and can greatly influence how care is perceived.[2] Hospitals that value, attract, and support exceptional people in these roles are making a crucial investment in person-centered care. When patients receive genuine empathy and respect, it not only improves their hospital experience but also supports their overall well-being and recovery.

Picker Principle: Involvement and Support for Family and Carers

It may not be standard practice for a world-renowned surgeon to call a family meeting before an operation. And if you're a surgeon reading this and throwing your hands up in the air in search of a reality check, I get it. But for us, Dr. Epstein's willingness to gather our family and walk us through what to expect made a tremendous difference. We entered surgery feeling more comfortable and informed, not just because we understood the medical details, but because Dr. Epstein's approach made the whole experience feel more human. He earned our trust and confidence from the very beginning, so much so that, even if things hadn't gone as hoped, we knew he had done everything possible for us.

Research supports the importance of the kind of interpersonal connection that Dr. Epstein established. A qualitative study found that when patients feel a strong connection and trust in their surgeon, they are more comfortable moving forward with surgery and more at ease with associated risks.[3] While the study focused on patient perspectives rather than the entire family, I believe my family's involvement contributed to the trust-building process and deepened our confidence during a stressful decision.

Opportunities for Person-Centered Care

Picker Principle: Attention to Physical and Environmental Needs

During my hospital stay, constipation became a significant challenge—one that's all too common for patients, especially those with limited mobility or on certain medications. Research shows that more than half of hospitalized patients experience constipation, yet it is often underrecognized and undertreated.[4] The standard medical solutions I was offered—enemas, suppositories, and various laxatives—were uncomfortable and invasive, and they only provided temporary relief.

Looking back, I wonder if a more proactive, holistic approach could have made a difference. Evidence now supports starting with non-pharmacological strategies, including ensuring adequate hydration, increasing fiber intake, and encouraging as much physical activity as possible. Simple dietary adjustments, such as adding more whole grains, fruits, and vegetables, and drinking plenty of water, can help prevent or relieve constipation and are recommended as first-line interventions.[5] These measures are not only less invasive but can also improve overall comfort and support recovery.

From a person-centered care perspective, addressing physical needs means looking beyond the immediate medical issue to consider the whole patient's experience. This includes providing clear information about prevention, respecting patients' preferences for less-invasive options, and creating an environment where patients feel comfortable discussing sensitive issues, such as bowel health. Addressing this secondary condition would have made my experience more tolerable and supported a smoother recovery.

Picker Principle: Clear Information, Communication, and Support for Self-Care

Losing bowel control wasn't a concern, but bladder function was an entirely different story, especially when it came to traveling on an airplane. Research indicates that many people use absorbent products such as disposable briefs or pads successfully, but intermittent catheterization may better meet the needs of some individuals with nerve-related bladder dysfunction during travel or when access to care is limited.[6]

I didn't fully appreciate the catheter option at the time, and I was fully prepared to just "diaper-up" and hope those TV ads about reliable and discreet disposable briefs weren't exaggerating. What I didn't consider was how much context matters. In the hospital, I'd had the support of trained professionals just a call button away. Traveling from the hospital to the airport, sitting on a plane for hours, and then riding to a new facility without access to personal care support was a completely different scenario. Ultimately, the decision was swayed not by my medical team, but by my hospital roommate (aka "my bonus nurse"). This experience highlighted the importance of healthcare providers (who are part of your medical team, not just sharing your room) providing clear, practical information that accounts for real-world circumstances. This empowers patients to make choices that improve comfort and that fit their lives outside of the hospital walls.

Picker Principle: Involvement in Decisions and Respect for Preferences

Agreeing to an optional catheterization is a bit like agreeing to an ice bath. Both might be good for you, but neither is something you look forward to. And while it may seem like I'm fixated on bladder and bowel function, "number one" and "number two" quickly became my number one and number two priorities.

My experiences with choices around catheterization highlight the nuances of the principle "involvement in decisions and respect for preferences." I was given the option to refuse routine catheterization in the hospital, and I was also presented with catheterization as an option for travel. However, in both cases, my medical team did not explain the reasons behind the recommendation. As a result, I was technically involved in the decision, and my preferences were honored, but the process lacked the depth and clarity it could have had if I had been given more information. Sometimes, a little extra context can make all the difference, ensuring that patient choices are truly informed and that care aligns with both best practices and individual needs.

My own situation did not involve religious or spiritual concerns, but I recognize how important these factors can be for others. Faith is a consideration for some when receiving care—like Muslim patients who may need space and time for daily prayer, or Orthodox Jews who refrain from medical treatment on the Sabbath. A comparative study of Jewish and Muslim patients notes that over-looking these religious needs can lead to ethical dilemmas, as both groups often rely on religious law and guidance from faith leaders in making medical decisions.[7] This is a reminder that what might seem like "preferences" are actually essential aspects of identity and belief for some, and deserve to be respected as such.

While I don't speak from personal experience, I share these examples to show how essential it is for care teams to recognize and respect the full spectrum of patient needs.

These scenarios underscore the importance of the Picker Principle surrounding the need for involvement in decisions and respect for preferences. For many patients, these are not simply preferences but deeply held religious obligations that should only be adjusted under exceptional circumstances. This highlights why it's crucial for care teams to understand these needs and strive to honor them whenever possible—even in emergency situations where patient safety must remain the top priority. Ultimately, that's what the Picker Principle is about: not just giving patients a voice, but understanding the "why" behind their choices.

• • •

CONVERSATION STARTERS

Thinking about new strategies is fantastic, but the magic starts to happen when you voice your thoughts and hear from others. Here are a few conversation starters to get the dialogue going.

For Patients, Providers, and Payers

Reflecting on the narrative in this chapter, are there additional moments where Picker principles were exemplified or fell short?

For Patients

1. How comfortable are you with speaking up when you don't understand something about your care or when you

need your care to be provided differently because of your values, religious beliefs, communication needs, disability accommodation requirements, or other personal traits? What might help you feel more empowered to ask questions or advocate for care that respects your needs?

2. How do you handle situations when you feel embarrassed or vulnerable during medical care? What strategies could help you overcome these feelings?

3. Think about your all-time favorite nursing assistant, nurse, doctor, or other healthcare provider. What stood out about them? What impact did they have on your experience? How did they know they had made a difference in your life?

4. How do you recognize when your support system (family, friends, caregivers) might be experiencing burnout? What could you do to support them?

For Providers

1. How do you identify when a patient's values, religious beliefs, communication needs, disability accommodations, or other personal factors require a different approach to care? How does your ability to recognize and respond to these needs affect the quality of care you provide? What strategies or resources help you meet these personal needs, and where do you see room for improvement in your practice?

2. What methods do you use to detect when patients might be withholding important information that could impact their care? How do you encourage them to share openly?

3. When working with patients, how do you avoid assumptions about their understanding of treatment? What techniques do you use to check for comprehension and invite questions or clarifications? How do you ensure patients understand why you're asking certain questions, so they can provide information that reflects their lifestyle and healthcare needs?

4. Reflecting on your current practices, how do you want your patients to remember you years from now? What specific, intentional actions or small changes can you implement today to help ensure their experience aligns with that legacy, even with time constraints?

For Payers

1. Prior authorization and network design are often described as evidence-based, but rare conditions, specialized needs, and underrepresented groups are sometimes left out of datasets. How does your organization evaluate and adjust policies and algorithms to prevent unintended denials or delays for patients who require exceptions, whether for clinical, cultural, linguistic, or religious reasons?

2. How do algorithms impact the quality of care offered to members, especially if they prioritize cost over medical necessity?

3. What processes are in place to review algorithms for fairness across all backgrounds and ensure decisions meet transparency standards?

4. How can your organization support employees in making coverage decisions, such as those related to prior

authorization or formulary approvals, in ways that reflect person-centered care principles? How might this include consideration of cultural and religious beliefs, disability accommodations, and patient-reported needs, while also ensuring that algorithm-informed processes or network limitations do not unintentionally overlook individual circumstances?

FOUR

INPATIENT REHAB

TEARS OF JOY (BUT MOSTLY PAIN)

My third and final hospital was in Detroit and about a twenty-minute drive from my parents' house in Southfield. With the major health crisis behind us, my focus shifted to learning how to walk again and mastering daily activities. The facility specialized in rehabilitation, and I received physical and occupational therapy five days a week, along with occasional recreational therapy. My physical therapy plan focused on strength building, balance, and walking. The occupational therapy focused on muscle coordination and activities of daily living. The purpose of recreational therapy was never really explained to me. I just remember having fun and other people to talk to. To round this out, I was still in a hospital setting, which meant I continued to receive the medical attention I needed.

Once I arrived at the hospital, the first order of business was removing the catheter. That was quick, easy, and painless. Next came inspecting my incision. It's never a good sign when your doctor uses noises to describe what he sees instead of words.

It turned out that my surgical incision was infected. But it wasn't the kind of infection that a dab of Neosporin could fix. The doctor had to open the infected skin with a scalpel, clean it with a solution, pack it with gauze, and cover it with protective tape to help it heal from the inside out. And that was just the beginning. To treat the infection, they had to insert a PICC line—a thin tube placed in a vein in my arm—to deliver strong antibiotics directly into my bloodstream. This approach is often used when infections require a stronger treatment than oral antibiotics (or a mother's kiss) can provide.

That part was especially tough. The idea of having a wound opened and packed with gauze made my skin crawl. What really got me was the wound care routine, which a nurse had to administer twice a day. First of all, just the thought of the nurse removing and stuffing gauze in the hole in my back made me feel like a stuffed animal. Think Build-A-Bear Workshop, but with fewer options and a lot more gauze. Then, there was the cold cleaning solution, which was like getting sprayed with a fire hose in the middle of winter. It didn't really hurt that much. Okay, it actually didn't hurt at all. But I pretended it did to encourage the nurse to speed things up. The whole process was so unpleasant that my mother was happy that I was in the hospital and not at home because she didn't have the stomach to perform that kind of wound care.

What was painful, though, was the PICC line with antibiotics. Looking back, that might have been my punishment for pretending to be in pain during the wound cleaning. The universe delivered on its threat to give me something to "cry about." The antibiotics burned so badly that it felt like acid running through my veins. The pain continued for days during the antibiotic treatment, until a new doctor visited me. Once I told him about the problem, he changed the antibiotic, and it made all the difference in the world.

The world of physical, occupational, and recreational therapy was still relatively new to me. Even though I had a physical therapist visit me for sessions in my New York hospital room, I didn't know what to expect in a large facility. But I knew I'd be able to get out of the hospital room, a luxury I didn't have in New York, so I was ready to go with the flow.

My physical therapy sessions took place in a large gym, full of treatment tables, mats, parallel bars for balancing, TheraBands, little steps that didn't lead anywhere, and lots of mirrors on the walls. The only things missing were TV screens and a smoothie bar.

The therapists at the facility pushed me to my limits, and a lot of pain was involved. There were times when I asked to go back to my room because I was in so much pain, but they always countered with a five-minute break and a cup of water. And you know what? That's all I ever needed.

I wasn't the only one who struggled in physical therapy. I found out that a former mayor of Detroit, a man renowned for his sharp tongue and intimidating personality, was in the very same facility. To give you a taste of his communication style, he once said, "Swearing is an art form. You can express yourself much more exactly, much more succinctly, with properly used curse words." When I asked the therapists what happened when he was in pain and wanted to go back to his room, the answer was just as exact and succinct. "He went back to his room."

Occupational therapy wasn't as physically daunting, but was just as important (especially since we got to bake brownies). The name makes it sound like they're preparing you to go to work, but in occupational therapy, "occupation" actually means the activities that *occupy* your day—things like bathing, getting dressed, cooking, and cleaning. Basically, occupational therapists help you relearn or adapt the skills you need to manage daily life.

The occupational therapy space was smaller than the physical therapy space. I did all types of activities to help with coordination. Throwing rings around cones, tossing beanbags in buckets, and knocking down a pyramid of cups with a beanbag. It was like being at a carnival with free games, but instead of winning prizes, you walked away with better balance and a competitive spirit.

But if you think occupational therapy is all fun and games, think again. These activities were just the warm-up to the main events, which involved all sorts of equipment that I'd never seen before. There was one machine that required you to pedal with your arms, like riding a bike for your upper body. Those exercises weren't exactly fun, but they were effective.

The occupational therapy room also had a kitchen, where we practiced cooking. Seeing a full kitchen in a rehabilitation space was an unexpected surprise for a newbie like me. It felt a bit like walking into a kitchen display at Ikea, except the oven turned on, the sink worked, and there was food in the refrigerator. Brownies aside, learning safety strategies to navigate kitchen hazards was really important for me, since I had weakness in my legs and balance issues.

The sessions for occupational therapy weren't just limited to that one room. Early in my stay, a therapist came to my room to help me shower and wash my hair. It was the first time I'd been able to get clean outside of my bed in weeks. She rolled me into the bathroom and helped me into a shower chair using a transfer board. She seemed confident about handling the shower itself, but when it came to washing my hair, she hesitated.

I can't recall her exact words, but I do remember that she let me take the lead. She watched as I worked through my routine—scrubbing my hair with shampoo, rinsing, repeating, applying conditioner, running a wide-tooth comb through my tight coils, and finishing with one last rinse. She seemed genuinely fascinated, especially when I sectioned my hair and started a French braid on each side. I had a feeling she was mentally taking notes, maybe for the next patient with thick hair texture similar to mine.

I loved my physical and occupational therapists, but the most enjoyable therapy I experienced was recreational therapy. I didn't get to go to recreational therapy on a daily basis, which may have made my time there all the more meaningful. We did a lot of craft projects, like making reindeer Christmas ornaments out of painted puzzle pieces. Yes, it may seem odd for a twenty-six-year-old to be excited about a craft project made from puzzle pieces. But when you live in a time with no streaming services, no smartphones, and no internet access, puzzle pieces and a little paint can turn an afternoon into something magical.

Once, we even got to take a field trip to the mall (except I was the one who got to sign the permission slip). After weeks of being in an institution, getting out into the fresh air felt amazing. Admittedly, things got a bit awkward when we were in the parking lot and I was on the lift of the wheelchair van. I spotted a woman staring at me, looking like she was about to cry. I felt bad for her because she felt bad for me, even though I was feeling pretty good. I actually wanted to reassure her that everything was okay. I think compassion is innate, and I never want to criticize anyone for feeling empathy. But sometimes, a lack of understanding can make people feel sorry for things that don't actually require pity. But that was a lesson for another day, because there was a frozen yogurt in the mall with my name on it.

Because I was back in my hometown of Detroit, my room was filled with visits from family and friends who brought lots of treats —mostly candy. Seeing them made me feel good, but bringing me treats made *them* feel good. Moderation isn't my strength, and I ate and ate and ate. Eventually, I had to do the unthinkable and ask people to stop bringing candy.

My mother visited during the day, and my dad would stop by most evenings after work. I quickly progressed enough to stand and take a few steps, so the staff trained my father to help me walk the hospital halls. He used a safety belt around my waist while I clung to the wall railing. I sort of felt like a dog being walked, but I didn't care. I was back on my feet (even if barely) and spending time with my dad, just like when I was a child.

With Christmas approaching, I really wanted to go home to be with my family. I'd already spent Halloween in the first hospital and Thanksgiving in the second, but Christmas was different. It was the holiday when everyone from my mother's side of the family (blood-related or not) gathered together. It was our social event of the year. My parents asked the hospital staff if they could check me out for a few hours, with my mother explaining that she would be hosting dinner at our home and was totally prepared to accommodate my needs. The staff agreed, and I got to go home for Christmas.

Under typical circumstances, the holidays can be overwhelming. But that Christmas gave me a whole new appreciation for being surrounded by loved ones. Everyone was happy to see me, and before heading back to the hospital, I even managed to walk a few steps. That was a real crowd-pleaser. It was like dancing down a *Soul Train* line, with everyone cheering, "Go, Cyn! Go, Cyn!" If you've never seen a Soul Train line, just picture two rows of people facing each other, grooving to the music, while others dance down the middle, and everyone cheers them on. Or better yet, look it up on YouTube.

Overall, I received excellent care at the third hospital—except for the few times I didn't. There was one instance where two nursing assistants transferred me from my wheelchair to the bed, with one bracing me under my arms and the other holding my legs. It felt like the one supporting my arms threw me on the bed like a sack of potatoes. I was in disbelief and asked myself: *Did that really happen?* I felt my suspicion was confirmed after he came back to apologize, which may have been prompted by his colleague.

On another occasion, a wheelchair attendant transported me from physical therapy back to my room. I had to go to the bathroom, but he was not trained or authorized to help with this. As always, I pressed the call button for assistance. After waiting for what seemed to be an eternity, an attendant entered my room. Although she didn't have authorization to offer bathroom support, she did have authorization to push my wheelchair. She took it upon herself to roll me to the nursing station and positioned me right next to the nurse, who was in the middle of telling a personal story to his colleagues. I'm sure he knew I'd called for him because he didn't ask what I needed. He just got up, rolled me back to my room, and helped me to the bathroom.

I can't say for certain what motivated these lapses in care, but I sometimes wondered if other factors were at play, perhaps rooted in preconceived notions, whether intentional or not. I've since learned that many patients with backgrounds similar to mine have had the same questions. Whether it's a one-off oversight or something more complicated, these moments linger and shape how you experience care.

Then there were moments that had nothing to do with assumptions or attitudes—like the nurse who honored my request for a later physical therapy start time but then announced for everyone to hear that I had "special grooming needs." For the record, that just meant I wanted time to wash up and do something with my hair so I didn't look like a hot mess.

Then there were the nursing students, who were learning how to draw blood. I felt lucky to have an expert like Dr. Epstein, so I never turned away a student who needed to practice. Now, to give context around blood withdrawal from my body, the inside of my arm is beige, and my veins are thick and dark green—so dark and juicy they should have been impossible to miss. But somehow, those nursing students managed to make drawing blood hurt. I mean, if I had classified secrets, I would have started talking. Still, letting them practice felt like my small contribution to the future of healthcare. Quality care has to start somewhere, so I figured I'd take one for the team.

As unpleasant as these instances were, the most challenging part of being in the third facility was when I had an emotional break-down. I thought I was being so strong by holding it together in front of everyone, even though there were many times when feeling confined and isolated had me down. But this one time, when my mother was leaving for the day, I could no longer stand the thought of being there, and I burst into tears. I kept saying over and over again, "I just want to go home." Of course, she felt bad because I was crying, but there was little she could do but try to console me.

Even with that episode, I remained grateful for the care, and when the therapists and doctors were able to negotiate with the insurance company for me to stay an extra week, I was happy to do so.

At the time, my hospital roommate was a woman I guessed to be in her sixties. She seemed nice, but we didn't talk much. Privacy was pretty loose back then. Having a "private" conversation just meant pulling the curtain. Because of that, we learned a lot about each other.

I once overheard a social worker discussing my roommate's discharge plans. Her husband was struggling with substance use, and there was uncertainty about whether she'd be able to go home or would need to move to a nursing facility. I knew all of this simply because we shared a room.

Those conversations made me realize she was being offered social work support. Because of relaxed privacy practices, I realized that I never received that kind of outreach. It was obvious that I had strong family support and a safe place to go after discharge. But if a social worker had checked in on me as well, I might have learned about resources or support to guide me through the emotional adjustments of recovery.

Instead, I was left to figure things out on my own.

When it was time for my discharge, I was over the moon. I was so ready to get out of that facility that I actually got a little arrogant. Back then, you'd receive your little menus and circle the options you wanted to eat for breakfast, lunch, and dinner. So when they came to give me my little piece of paper the night before discharge, I told them, "No thanks." My parents were coming in the morning, and I wouldn't be around for breakfast (see ya!).

I woke up with everything packed and ready to go. As I waited in bed, the food services staff were making their rounds with breakfast delivery. The lady assigned to my floor was kind enough to offer me a tray, even though I hadn't completed the little form the night before.

"No, I'm good," I told her. "My parents will be here any minute. Thanks."

We didn't have cell phones back then, but I did have a telephone in my hospital room. Since I hadn't gotten a call about a delay, I figured they'd be there any minute. I started browsing what was on television, which didn't take long, with only five channels to choose from. I landed on the movie *Seven Brides for Seven Brothers*. I wasn't going to be there long enough to watch the entire movie. I just needed something to keep me company until my parents showed up.

By the time the closing credits rolled, food services came around with lunch. At that point, the arrogance that I'd felt that morning had turned into confusion. *Did they forget that I was getting out today, or did I just get stood up?* The food services attendant offered me a lunch tray. I tried to maintain my composure, but I wasn't nearly as confident this time around. "Ah, no. My family will be here any minute." She looked at me with a little sympathy, almost like she was holding on to some inside information.

By mid-afternoon, I felt like the last kid waiting to be picked up from school, except there was no teacher stuck there to supervise me—just the food services lady who'd seen this scene play out a hundred times before. All of the frustration I'd felt during those long hours melted away the moment my mother walked through the door. Turns out my parents were retrofitting the house just right to make me as comfortable as possible, and it just took a lot longer than they'd expected.

I was finally going home.

• ● •

PERSON-CENTERED CARE DISCUSSION

Reflecting on Rehab

I witnessed many moments of clinical excellence and genuine compassion during rehab, as well as a few bumps along the way.

Here's where my experience aligned with person-centered care—and where it missed the mark.

Alignment With Person-Centered Care

Picker Principle: Effective Treatment by Trusted Professionals

The quality of care I received at the rehabilitation facility was excellent and reflected person-centered care principles. My physical therapists skillfully balanced evidence-based practices with attention to my individual needs. For instance, when I felt pain and wanted to return to my room, the staff didn't just give me a simple yes or no. Instead, they addressed the underlying problem, which was my discomfort. Offering me space to regroup allowed me to feel better and continue with the therapy I needed to recover. It felt so reasonable that I didn't even realize I was involved in a negotiation. Their approach built trust and made me feel seen. Helping me get through the treatment in a way that worked for me positioned my care team to advocate for an extra week of therapy—a request that the insurance company approved.

Research in physical therapy settings highlights that mutual respect, shared decision-making, and two-way communication between patients and physical therapists help foster stronger therapeutic relationships and improve patient engagement.[1] Person-centered care isn't just about the clinical treatment. It's about understanding what drives patients and developing strategies that will help them benefit from clinical expertise. Feeling heard and supported helped me engage more effectively in my care, leading to a more positive rehabilitation experience and an extra week of treatment.

Picker Principle: Involvement and Support for Family and Carers

While my parents were always supportive and involved in decisions, it was at the rehabilitation facility that their role became truly transformative. There, they shifted from playing an active role in decision-making to serving as "deputy healthcare providers." Learning best practices to help me develop practical skills, like safely walking me down the hall using a special belt, contributed to my recovery and prepared me for life after discharge.

The facility provided the professional expertise, while my family's understanding of my personality and what motivated me kept me engaged and encouraged me to push further. My experience is consistent with research findings. One qualitative study found that when family members are actively involved in rehabilitation, their unique insights into the patient's personality, routines, and subtle changes can inform clinical decisions, support patient safety, and promote engagement in recovery.[2]

This collaboration ensured that my care didn't end at the facility's doors. By combining professional guidance with personal insight, the rehabilitation team empowered my family to play a meaningful role in my healing process.

Picker Principle: Clear Information, Communication, and Support for Self-Care

The quality of care at the rehabilitation facility stood out largely because of the staff's ability to foster open communication that went both ways and support my self-care. This involved a lot of listening (not just waiting for me to stop talking) and developing strategies that aligned with my interests. Their approach helped get at the root of my concerns, whether it was the pain caused by the PICC line, the discomfort from physical therapy, or my desire to go home for Christmas.

But observing also upheld this principle, which is exactly what happened when the occupational therapist realized that the best thing she could do for me (and probably for herself) was to watch and learn as I went through my haircare routine. By realizing her limitations, she demonstrated humility and willingness to learn from me, while honoring my dignity and cultural identity.

My occupational therapist was ahead of her time. Cultural humility is increasingly recognized in healthcare as essential for building trust and improving communication. It emphasizes ongoing self-reflection, recognition of power dynamics, and accountability in building respectful and responsive relationships with patients, which ultimately contributes to better health outcomes.[3]

The way that most of the staff engaged with me, whether they were listening, conveying information, or observing, demonstrated how true person-centered care respects and responds to the whole person as a unique individual, not just a case.

Opportunities for Person-Centered Care

Picker Principle: Continuity of Care and Smooth Transitions

My experience transitioning from the New York hospital to the rehabilitation facility in Detroit demonstrated the critical importance of continuity of care and smooth transitions in achieving person-centered care. In my case, an infected incision led to a secondary health issue that required an aggressive and painful treatment plan. Fortunately, once the care team identified the source of my pain and switched my antibiotic, the discomfort subsided, which goes to show how responsive adjustments can make all the difference.

Even small oversights during a care transition, like gaps in communication, medication management, or follow-up, can lead to significant problems after discharge.[4] The good news is that comprehensive discharge planning and effective information transfer between care settings significantly reduce readmission rates and improve patient outcomes.[5]

Every single system has the opportunity to evolve, especially those meant to protect patients. The Picker Principle on continuity of care and smooth transitions helps care teams ensure safe handoffs and discharges, support patient health, and equip future providers with the information they need to deliver the best possible care.

Picker Principle: Emotional Support, Empathy, and Respect

My entire ordeal was a rollercoaster of emotions that began well before I arrived at the rehabilitation hospital. Early on, I was afraid that I might die, but after the surgery, those fears were replaced by the emotional toll of a long hospital stay. And it was this third hospital where I reached my breaking point.

The emotional strain felt just as intense as my physical pain, but those emotional needs were invisible and went unacknowledged. Since no one brought it up, neither did I. I didn't realize until much later that even with excellent healthcare, the emotional challenges can be just as demanding as the physical ones.

My experience isn't unique. One literature review found that hospitalized patients frequently experience depression, anxiety, and emotional distress, and that these psychological effects are often under-recognized and inadequately addressed by healthcare providers.[6]

The gap between physical care and emotional support reinforces a vital truth: a diagnosis is just one part of a person, and real care means seeing, centering, and supporting the whole person.

Picker Principle: Attention to Physical and Environmental Needs

Attending to patients' physical and environmental needs is a fundamental pillar of quality healthcare, and safety is central to that effort. In clinical settings, safety means making sure patients receive the correct medications, are protected from falls or injuries, and are cared for in a clean, hygienic environment that supports healing. These are just a few of the many important factors that contribute to a comprehensive approach to patient safety. And that's just the beginning. For the most part, my experience aligned with this Picker principle. But when it was overlooked, the impact was significant and lasting.

The most glaring example came when the nursing assistant roughly tossed me onto the bed, despite my infected incision and physical vulnerability. Even with only one other person in the room, it was humiliating. And that's saying something—after being bathed, given suppositories, and placed on bedpans by strangers, that moment was the only time I truly felt humiliated during my hospital stay.

Another moment that stayed with me didn't rise to the level of humiliation, but it was still deeply uncomfortable. A nurse chose to keep socializing with colleagues rather than help me to the bathroom. This wasn't just frustrating; delaying access to toileting assistance can increase the risk of complications, like a bladder infection.

As disappointing as those two situations were, what lingers most is the fact that I didn't speak up. I don't know if it was shame, uncertainty about how to report it, or some deeply ingrained "snitches get stitches" mindset. Maybe it was a combination of all three. But what I do know is that I'm not alone. A Joint Commission report identifies patient reluctance to speak up as a system-wide issue embedded in healthcare culture and communication barriers. It calls on healthcare organizations to foster trust, clarify reporting processes, and empower patients to voice concerns without fear—key steps toward safer, more equitable, and higher-quality care.[7]

In one situation, I witnessed a colleague step in to make things better; in another, I suspect someone quietly intervened behind the scenes. These moments demonstrate the importance of empowering employees to speak up or take action when something isn't right. Even when such efforts go unrecognized or unrewarded, they reflect a deep commitment to high-quality care, and the value of having people who take genuine pride in their work.

● ● ●

CONVERSATION STARTERS

Whether you've received care, helped deliver it, or supported others behind the scenes, these questions are meant to inspire thoughtful conversations about your personal or professional experiences.

For Patients, Providers, and Payers

Reflecting on the narrative in this chapter, are there additional moments where Picker principles were exemplified or fell short?

For Patients

1. What helps you feel safe in a healthcare facility? If something in your environment didn't feel safe, would you feel comfortable speaking up? What impact could patient feedback have on creating a safer environment?

2. What's required for good support after leaving a medical facility? For example, clear communication, emotional support, coordinated follow-up, or access to resources. What matters most to you, and why?

3. What efforts have you noticed in healthcare facilities to respect your privacy, whether through the environment or in how patient information is handled? Why is this important, and where are there opportunities to strengthen privacy?

4. Have you experienced pain when receiving care? How did your healthcare provider work with you to resolve the issue? If there were no safe medical options for relief without compromising care, was this explained to you? Is there anything you wish you had done differently?

For Providers

1. What measures are in place to ensure patient safety? How do you empower staff and patients to speak up

when safety may be compromised, and what protections are in place to prevent retaliation?

2. Do the protocols at your facility effectively support smooth transitions and information sharing? What has worked well, and where have you seen opportunities for improvement?

3. What types of psychosocial or emotional support does your facility offer patients and families, and how are they informed about these resources? Is this information provided to everyone?

4. How do you involve family members, friends, or other support individuals identified by the patient in the care process to enhance communication, reinforce education, and improve safety outcomes?

For Payers

1. How do you ensure that patients have prompt access to specialized services—including extensions of care when clinically necessary—without unnecessary delays or administrative barriers?

2. How do you evaluate and support the provision of psychosocial and emotional health services in rehabilitation and other settings, and are these services covered as part of the standard benefit package?

3. What mechanisms exist for patients and families to appeal or request reconsideration when they feel their care needs, such as extended rehabilitation or specialized therapies, are not being fully met under their current coverage?

4. How does your organization monitor and address patient experiences of dignity, privacy, and respect, especially during transitions of care in contracted facilities? What systems ensure warm handoffs between providers, and how do you use patient concerns to drive system-wide quality and culture improvements, rather than relying on individual discipline alone?

"Disability doesn't make you exceptional, but questioning what you think you know about it does."
—Attributed to Stella Young

PART B: ELEVATOR DREAMS

THE (NOT SO) FINE PRINT ABOUT PART B

The first four chapters followed my hospital journey. But after discharge, my healthcare experience became less linear and more layered, stretching beyond clinical care into community living. Over twenty-five-plus years, I've navigated outpatient therapy, embraced a new disability identity, accessed social services, returned to school, and pursued vocational rehab—mostly through trial and error.

Because my experiences after discharge are hard to capture in a straight timeline, I organize Part B by topic, using headers that reflect different aspects of my journey. Along the way, social drivers of health, like housing, education, transportation, community resources, and family support, emerged as important factors that shaped my health outcomes and my life.

Chapters 5–7 explore:

- Adjusting to my environment and disability identity
- Support from family, friends, and government programs

- Medicine, provider assumptions, and medical advancements

Using the National Advisory Board's (NAB) Six Principles to Modernize the Healthcare Infrastructure, I highlight examples that show how my experience fits this framework—and how systemic change is still needed. Each chapter ends with conversation starters for patients, providers, and payers working to make person-centered care a reality beyond clinic walls. I continue to use the word "patient" in this context because, even as the setting shifts from healthcare facility to home, engagement with healthcare professionals and systems remains.

FIVE

NEW BODY, "WHO DIS?"

TRANSITIONING INTO DISABILITY

Being discharged from the hospital was a huge milestone in my recovery, but it was far from the finish line. I found myself facing a new reality, one that involved adjusting to my new body and navigating my new identity as a person with a disability. Here's what that experience was like.

PHYSICAL ADJUSTMENT: WELCOME TO YOUR NEW REALITY

As much as I valued my independence before the surgery, I was happy to return to my parents' house after leaving the third and final hospital. This relief hit me as soon as I got home. Even though I had the privilege of receiving top-notch care, the feeling of being "institutionalized," if only for a few weeks, was confining. Finally, I was free from the rigid schedule dictating when I woke up, had blood work and vitals taken, ate, and went to therapy. Freedom, home cooking, and the company of my family—this was good living.

It wasn't long before I realized that even with my newfound freedom, I still needed just as much support from my parents as I did when I lived there as a child. After all, I could only walk a few steps on my own. I needed help with bathing and basic household chores, and I couldn't cook a full meal by myself. The doctors told me that my walking would improve with physical therapy over the next year, but that I'd plateau twelve to eighteen months after the surgery, so I had a lot of work to do.

My parents lived in a two-story home where all the bedrooms were on the second floor. Instead of moving me back into my childhood room, they retrofitted the bedroom that had been converted into an office because it was closest to the staircase. They reshuffled furniture from the other rooms to make space. When I returned from the hospital, it contained only a bed, a chair, and a nightstand, making it easier for me to navigate.

I slept upstairs and made one trip downstairs each day. Every morning, I'd scoot down the steps on my backside, a skill I'd perfected as a child. Once I reached the bottom, I lifted myself up on the banister and grabbed onto my red walker that was always there waiting for me. It was fully loaded with wheels, handbrakes, a basket, and a little seat so I could sit whenever I got tired. Using it reminded me of the car Fred Flintstone drove during the opening credits, except I had to stand to operate it. Outside of the house, I used a wheelchair that was pretty lightweight, making it relatively easy for people driving me around to get it in and out of the trunk. My insurance company covered both devices.

Even with my fancy equipment, it was really hard getting around the house, but I acted like everything was just fine. Since I was alone during the day, I was terrified that my parents would put me in adult daycare (now commonly referred to as "adult day services"). I didn't even really know what adult daycare was. I just knew that I couldn't take being in another facility.

"Oh, I'm great," I'd say. "I've got everything I need. You can go." In reality, during my first week at home I found myself sitting on the couch all day. While the house was updated to make getting around possible, we hadn't really tackled the realities of everyday living yet. Sometimes I thought about the amenities of hospital living. Recreational therapy gave me something fun to do. I had help getting to the bathroom. And meals were delivered right to my room.

Being home alone meant my only company was the television. Instead of getting help from an assistant, I relied on hopes and dreams to make it to the bathroom on time. And hospital room service was replaced with a microwave and some Domino's coupons.

So yes, I was happy to be home, but it didn't turn out to be the victory lap that I'd imagined. After all, I didn't have my own place, I wasn't earning any money, and I had no transportation. True independence was still out of reach.

THE GREAT ESCAPE:
GETTING BACK INTO THE COMMUNITY

It wasn't long until my outpatient physical therapy began. Yes, it was at a facility, but at least I was back with other people. Plus, when it was over, I got to go home instead of back to the hospital room. Since I couldn't drive, my mother made up a schedule for her friends and my aunts to help out with the transportation. We didn't live in an area known for mass transit, so it never occurred to us to look into accessible public transportation.

Around the same time, I also enrolled in the few classes I

needed to finish up my teaching certification. My mother had made sure I registered while I was still in the hospital, which left me a bit uneasy. Sure, I'd zipped around the hospital using a wheelchair without a problem, but on campus? Campus would be like an obstacle course with spectators. *How was I supposed to deal with that?* I thought.

When I called to register from my hospital bed, I actually thought I was going to get out of it. The man on the other end told me that I had to come down to campus to register (remember, this was before broad internet adoption), but I couldn't keep my mouth shut. When I explained my situation and that I wouldn't be out of the hospital in time to register, he registered me on the spot.

Before the classes began, my mother drove me to campus for a dry run to check for accessible entrances and routes, and she helped me navigate the building since I was still learning to manage a wheelchair outside of a hospital setting.

I didn't fully appreciate it at the time, but the Americans with Disabilities Act (ADA) made navigating campus and other spaces outside of my home so much easier. This legislation, which was passed in 1990, had only recently started to reshape public spaces when I became disabled. As a result of this act, new and altered public spaces had to provide accessible routes in most cases, often meaning elevators in multilevel buildings, curb cuts in sidewalks, and accessible parking spots.

While therapy helped me get back on my feet, it was probably enrolling in those classes that accelerated the process. One of the classes involved a trip to a children's museum built before the ADA that had a second floor and no elevator. When I asked how children who used wheelchairs managed to get to the second floor, I was told that the staff carried them up. Adjusting to my new reality as a wheelchair user was one thing, but unless it was

Lenny Kravitz doing the lifting, I was not getting carried up the steps.

I also couldn't stomach the thought of my classmates looking on as I used the scooching up the stairs on my butt method like I did at home. So, I worked really, really hard at physical therapy, and by the time we visited the museum a few months later, I was able to essentially pull myself up the steps using the handrail. Overall, the return to school and all of the environmental barriers that came with it were challenging, but they gave me a sense of purpose and connection that extended beyond my recovery routine.

SOFT LANDINGS SHOULDN'T BE A LUXURY

I eventually went from using my wheelchair to a walker, to a four-pronged cane, and finally to a straight cane. But since I was still in recovery, I had to leave my job. Thank goodness for COBRA, the federal law that lets you keep your employer-sponsored health insurance after leaving a job, which made my health coverage seamless. Back then, COBRA insurance seemed more affordable and straightforward than it does today.

Looking back on this time, I know my physical recovery would have been much different if I hadn't had a safe and supportive place to land after discharge. The combination of my family's unwavering support, access to the right equipment, and a home environment adapted to my needs made all the difference. That foundation allowed me to focus on healing and rebuilding my life in a way that felt right for me.

I also recognize that not everyone is as fortunate. Many people leave the hospital without a strong support system, adapted living spaces, or the resources needed to recover safely and independently. Social drivers of health, such as access to safe and affordable housing, reliable social networks, and community resources, play a crucial role in recovery. Too often, the difference between a smooth transition and ongoing struggle comes down to the presence or absence of these supports, which are influenced by broader social, economic, and environmental factors. Everyone deserves the chance to recover in an environment that meets their needs and is surrounded by people who can help them thrive.

IDENTITY ADJUSTMENT: THE MAKEOVER I WASN'T EXPECTING

Transitioning into disability was tough. I wish it had come with a manual. Understanding what I do about disability now, I'm sure I knew people with disabilities before that point—but I just didn't realize it. Disability as an identity just wasn't on my radar. I didn't even know I had a disability until I went to a follow-up appointment with a doctor, and she gave me paperwork for a disability parking tag. When she first brought it up, I was like, "Who is this for?" (which I asked from my wheelchair). It's not that I rejected the label of "disability," I just didn't know how it applied to me. I didn't know about disability. I didn't know anyone who identified as having a disability. And it never crossed my mind that I had a disability. I just knew my legs didn't work like they used to.

The doctor explained that my mobility was impaired and, even though I wasn't driving, I could still use the tag when I was a passenger in a car. When I realized I was eligible for one of those coveted parking spots, everything came into focus. That was how I came to understand that I was disabled. I actually got excited and thought, *Yeah, I have a disability. Where do I sign?*

The first time someone used a label to describe my disability in a social context didn't happen until years later. By then, I was walking with a cane and preparing to move into campus housing for the summer during my graduate program. Turns out there was a set of steps I hadn't anticipated when I signed the housing agreement.

When I explained my concerns to the woman working in the front office, she glanced at my cane and understood the issue. Wanting to help, she called the main housing office to advocate on my behalf, but the person on the other end didn't seem to grasp the problem. Growing frustrated, the woman finally blurted out, "This girl is crippled—she can't do these stairs!"

For those unfamiliar, *crippled* is an outdated term that doesn't land well in modern times.

Crippled? It felt like I'd stepped into a black-and-white movie from the '50s. I was torn. On one hand, I appreciated her fierce advocacy, but on the other, the word stung. After all, she was on a mission to get me out of the housing agreement, and as it turned out, that's exactly what she did.

Now, before you go clutching your pearls, I have to confess that I wasn't even up to par when it came to disability etiquette and language myself. I knew enough not to go around calling people "crippled." But I had always used the word "handicapped," not to describe people but to describe parking spots.

I'd also thought that the big stalls in restrooms were just for people to spread out. I learned firsthand that when you're a wheelchair user, you need to be able to transfer from the chair to the toilet, and the extra space, coupled with the handrails on the side, makes the process that much easier. So, gradually, I started replacing the adjective "handicapped" with "accessible." That can be challenging, though, because a lot of people don't know what I'm talking about when I say "accessible."

It's also tough for more personal reasons. Understanding that the word "handicapped" is so dated, I just don't want to use it when describing parking or bathroom stalls. I don't want to be out of touch like the woman who helped me with the housing. And I get so frustrated with myself when I do slip up, and I'm embarrassed when I'm around people who know I should know better. When this happens and I'm conscious of it, I quickly correct myself. I've never been shamed for this, but still, it doesn't feel good.

With so many nuances behind language and disability, I learned about person-first language (putting the person first) and identity-first language (referencing identity first). Everyone is different, but I actually go back and forth between "disabled" and "person with a disability." I'm really comfortable with both, but in my experience, I have found that a lot of people who have not personally experienced disability are cautious about these terms and use other terminology like "differently abled," "physically challenged," and "handi*capable*." I appreciate the concern about my self-esteem, but what I really want is a place to sit down.

Of course, not everyone in the disability community feels the same way. Some embrace these alternative terms, while others prefer more direct language like "disabled" or "person with a disability." My circle of friends with disabilities and I tend to chuckle or roll our eyes at those alternative terms. Some even take offense.

For the most part, I personally believe that these alternative terms are often offered in the spirit of sensitivity. But the real challenge isn't the word "disability" itself, but the stigma and discomfort society places around it. Instead of trying to avoid disability as an identity, I'd love for people to focus on challenging the stigma around disability and recognize it as a valid part of some people's experience as human beings.

IT'S OKAY TO LOOK, JUST DON'T FORGET TO BLINK

For me, the hardest part about transitioning into disability was the disconnect between how I saw myself and how my body *and* the world reacted to me. Mentally, I felt like the same person; only my circumstances had changed. Things were different in terms of how my body felt, though. It's hard to feel like the same person when your legs don't do what you want them to do, and you're in pain every minute of every day.

When it came to social situations, early on, when I used a wheelchair, I felt that people became uncomfortable around me, almost as if they were reminding themselves, *Don't look at the chair. Don't look at the chair.* Instead, they'd lock gazes with me and refuse to break eye contact, like they were magicians-in-training trying to hypnotize me and thought that my wheelchair might somehow break the spell of normal conversation. That intense focus made ordinary interactions feel strained and served as a constant reminder that there was something about me so obvious, yet treated by society as if it shouldn't be seen.

It wasn't until I became disabled that I truly appreciated just how many different types of disabilities exist. Some, like mine, are observable and immediately apparent. Others, such as cognitive or psychiatric disabilities, are less obvious. There are also health conditions and physical disabilities that may not be noticeable to others but can be just as impactful. The fact that a disability isn't immediately apparent doesn't make it any less significant or diminish the need for accommodations and understanding.

I recognize that, in some ways, I've been fortunate. Because my disability is noticeable, people often extend me grace if I'm walking more slowly or offer assistance when trying to navigate physical barriers. I know that many people with less noticeable disabilities don't always receive the same understanding, even though their challenges are just as real. This has made me even more aware of the importance of empathy and accommodation for all disabilities, whether you can see them or not.

I share this because we may not always understand someone else's experience or identity, and that's okay. We don't have to "figure someone out" to treat them with respect and empathy. Sometimes, it's enough to accept that a stranger's story is different from our own, and that's perfectly okay.

• • •

PERSON-CENTERED CARE DISCUSSION

Transitioning Into Disability

Given the focus on transitioning into disability in home and community settings, I draw on the Six Principles to Modernize the Healthcare Infrastructure developed by the National Advisory Board (NAB) on Improving Healthcare Services for Older Adults and People with Disabilities. Here's how the early part of my transition into disability aligned with and deviated from these principles.

Alignment With Person-Centered Care

NAB Principle: Improve Health and Well-being Through Individual Empowerment and System Coordination

My transition home after surgery was shaped by coordination between my care team, family, and insurance provider. This began before discharge, when my care team identified the type of outpatient physical therapy I would need, along with a wheelchair and walker. They also guided my family in retrofitting our home for accessibility to support my safety and independence. Even though I was no longer under the hospital's direct care, this intentional planning meant my family and I weren't left to navigate recovery alone.

My experience mirrors research showing that effective transitional care that is rooted in close coordination among providers, patients, and families through discharge planning, caregiver preparation, and follow-up support is linked to better outcomes and greater patient independence during recovery.[1]

The benefits of this coordinated and empowering approach extended beyond physical progress—it gave me the confidence I needed as I moved forward to reimagine and rebuild my life. My experience brings to life the NAB principle that improving health and well-being benefits from both individual empowerment and system coordination. When providers, patients, families, and payers work in alignment, they lay the foundation for a successful recovery.

NAB Principle: Achieve Community Inclusion and Full Participation

Without a doubt, the ADA was essential for community inclusion and full participation. Before my injury, the ADA was just an abstract law I'd heard about in passing, but once I began using a wheelchair, it became my ticket to independence. But the law isn't a magic wand. Despite its promise, gaps in implementation remain—from inconsistent physical accessibility in public buildings and transit to uneven adoption of accessibility policies and ongoing barriers to mental healthcare and public services.[2] While full implementation is essential to realize the ADA's potential, I still credit the legislation with enabling me to experience the NAB principle involving community inclusion and full participation.

Opportunities for Person-Centered Care

NAB Principle: Achieve Access to Meaningful Work and Activities

When I first returned home after the hospital, I wasn't ready to go back to work. But looking back, I probably would have benefited from faster access to meaningful activities involving recreation and social engagement.

While outpatient therapy and classes provided some interaction, they focused on recovery and academics rather than fun, hobbies, or community connection. At the time, options for connecting with others outside the home were limited. The need to coordinate transportation made it difficult to leave the house at will, and online discussion forums were rare since the internet was just starting to gain traction. As a result, there was no easy way to connect with others, making it even harder to participate in community life or find peer support beyond my immediate circle.

I wish I'd known about the Centers for Independent Living when I was discharged from rehab. They may have helped with transportation resources, recreational programs, peer support, or referrals to accessible activities sooner. Access to these types of opportunities offered through Centers for Independent Living can go a long way toward developing a sense of purpose and belonging. As important as this support is, many people are left out because there isn't a center nearby, which amplifies a critical gap in access to community support.

The absence of meaningful social engagement is associated with health consequences. Research indicates that adults who lack social support after hospital discharge have a greater risk of rehospitalization.[3]

Alignment with the NAB principle means ensuring that people with disabilities have real choices and support to participate fully in valued roles and activities—not just in work, but in all aspects of community life. Access to meaningful activities could have supported my mental health, nurtured my social connections, and helped me transition from just trying to make it through the day to truly thriving.

NAB Principle: Value Dignity and Choice

I'm a little embarrassed to admit this, but my transition into disability challenged my sense of dignity in ways I hadn't anticipated. Before my spinal cord surgery, I was part of what I now call the "straight-walking community"—those who move through the world without thinking twice about their walking pattern. Suddenly, I was navigating a new identity, and I was unsure how to process my feelings or where to turn for support. No one directly denied me dignity, but I didn't have the information needed to feel empowered in my new circumstances.

Without guidance or connection to disability culture and community, I carried unnecessary fears about venturing outside the hospital, the only other place where I felt understood and accepted outside of my parents' home. After discharge, I hid my struggles because I worried that admitting to them might mean losing more control over my life by being sent to another institution. This left me feeling isolated, making those early days far more difficult than they needed to be.

I recently discovered a body of scholarship on disability identity development that describes four key areas people may experience or revisit throughout their lives: acceptance, building relationships within the disability community, adopting shared values, and engaging with the community at large.[4]

Here's how this framework applies to me:

- *Acceptance:* Coming to terms with my new reality was not immediate. My ongoing efforts to "walk smoother" over the years suggest that for me, acceptance was a gradual process.
- *Building Relationships:* It wasn't until about two years post-surgery, when I began volunteering at a Center for Independent Living, that I started forming meaningful connections within the disability community.
- *Adopting Shared Values:* My scholarship on accessible technology introduced me to the broader values of the disability community like pride, advocacy, and the understanding that disability is a natural part of the human experience.
- *Engaging with the Community at Large:* Moving out of my parents' house for graduate school marked my first real step toward independently engaging with the wider world. It helped me begin to reestablish a sense of independence.

This framework acknowledges that disability identity development is not linear but fluid and shaped by broader social and cultural contexts. Although I didn't have this insight earlier, knowing that my journey follows a path recognized by others brings clarity and comfort. A simple "trust the process" might have eased some of the emotional burden, offering much-needed relief.

The NAB principle emphasizes dignity and choice in long-term services and supports, but those values also apply to disability identity development. Each phase—acceptance, connection, shared values, and engagement—requires support that fosters confidence and self-determination. Early on, I struggled without guidance. That gap reveals a broader need to support identity, not just function, in truly person-centered care.

• • •

CONVERSATION STARTERS

Whether you're navigating temporary challenges or permanent changes in functioning—either for yourself or someone you support —these questions can spark meaningful conversations about support during important transitions.

For Patients, Providers, and Payers

Reflecting on the narrative in this chapter, are there additional moments where NAB principles were exemplified or fell short?

For Patients

1. How have you adapted—both physically and emotionally—to changes in your health or function? What types of support or resources have helped you feel more confident and in control during this adjustment?

2. What physical, social, or emotional barriers can impact healthcare? What kinds of support—whether from people, policies, or services—could help address these challenges?

3. Which activities, like hobbies, spending time with friends, or work, matter most to you, and how might you stay involved, even if you need to adapt how you participate?

4. Consider a time when your health condition made it harder to do everyday activities. What adjustments did you make? How did they help, and where did they fall short? What might you do differently next time?

For Providers

1. How do you support patients and families as they adjust to changes in function, whether due to temporary conditions or permanent disability? What approaches help build confidence and adaptability during these transitions?

2. How do you support patients' evolving needs to help them maintain independence and quality of life within their communities as their functional abilities change, whether temporarily or permanently?

3. Do you feel confident about disability etiquette and engaging with patients with disabilities appropriately? When have you felt particularly effective, and when do you feel you could have done better?

4. Are you attentive to the emotional and identity-related aspects of disability, and do you create space for patients

to share concerns about stigma, language, or self-perception?

For Payers

1. How do your feedback systems help you understand and respond to the emotional needs of members whose health conditions affect their ability to participate in daily life?
2. How do you recognize and support the emotional, social, and practical challenges members face when adjusting to changes in health or transitioning into disability, including navigating financial and systemic barriers like complex paperwork or limited provider networks?
3. How do your policies ensure that home, community, or clinical environments are responsive to members' changing functional needs or evolving identities during health transitions?
4. How does your organization ensure that members experiencing significant physical changes receive adequate emotional and psychological support, particularly if there's a shortage of trained caregivers and mental health professionals? What steps do you take to connect patients with counseling, peer support, or community resources? How do you prepare care navigators and staff to identify and respond to these emotional needs effectively?

SIX

HELP DESK CENTRAL

FAMILY, SOCIAL SERVICES, AND
THE PAPERWORK OLYMPICS

Getting comfortable with my new body and evolving identity was like on-the-job training, but without the employee handbook or welcome swag. And adjusting to the new me was just the beginning.

Reentering society after my hospital stay felt a bit like waking up from a long nap. Think Rip Van Winkle, but with full consciousness. Somehow, everything had changed. I didn't recognize any of the music on the radio. Movies like *Titanic* were suddenly clocking in at over three hours. And more and more people were trading in their fax numbers for AOL email addresses.

I had to figure out how to navigate public spaces, piece together systems of support (which often felt like a scavenger hunt), and adapt to a world that suddenly seemed very different. What does this have to do with person-centered care? A truly person-centered approach recognizes that health is shaped not only by medical treatment, but also by the environments we navigate, the resources we can access, and the everyday challenges we face—all of which are social drivers of health. My family and I approached all of this without a guide, so I hope that by sharing my experience, I can help others facing similar challenges.

THE FRIENDS AND FAMILY DEAL

During my hospitalization, the nurses, nursing assistants, doctors, therapists, food services staff, and other hospital personnel were my primary caregivers. However, once I returned home, that responsibility shifted to my family.

I'm not sure if they ever sat down and mapped out a formal plan for my care, but their support was undeniably strategic. My parents divided responsibilities, welcomed help from friends and relatives, and ensured I remained accountable for my physical therapy, daily tasks, and future planning.

Caregiver fatigue is real, and this approach helped them avoid burnout. Plus, establishing expectations for me not only lightened their load but also spared me the guilt of feeling like a burden. Their expectations were empowering and gave me a sense of purpose and accomplishment.

My father assumed the role of captain of my in-home physical recovery. He'd tie a safety belt around my waist, as they'd taught him at the rehabilitation hospital, and hold on to it as we walked laps through the house together. The loop of connected rooms on the first floor made walking laps easy. We'd start in the foyer and then step into the living room (which was one of the few times my mother let us in there when we didn't have company). Then we'd enter the dining room and walk a short distance to the kitchen. Our last space was the family room before returning to the foyer. Granted, the lap was short, but these walks became a special bonding ritual for my father and me.

Now, I know this hasn't aged well, but when I was growing up, our family operated under traditional roles in many ways. My father handled repairs, took out the trash, and did the heavy lifting. My mother made sure the house was in tip-top shape and did the cooking, which meant my father was used to being served. When my mother wasn't around, I was the one doing the serving.

My walker and weak legs didn't change a thing. If my father wanted a bowl of ice cream, chips, or anything that could fit in the basket on my walker, I was expected to retrieve it. The one time I complained about having to serve him because of my mobility issues, he just told me, while barely glancing away from the television, that it was part of my physical therapy. As annoying as it was, I have to admit that these routines helped me regain a sense of stability and even a bit of independence.

In those early days, my father also took on the task of helping me in and out of the shower. It might sound awkward, but after being cared for by hospital staff, who handled all of my most personal needs (bathing, toileting, changing pads), having my father help me in this way didn't feel like a big deal. We had a routine: I'd wrap myself in a towel, he'd help me onto the shower chair, and I'd use a handheld spray in the shower. When I was done, I'd grab the towel (which hung within arm's reach), dry off, wrap myself up again, and call for him when I was ready to get out. Simple as that.

I never asked if it was awkward for him, but I imagine he was just so grateful I was alive that he welcomed the chance to help.

My mother became the designated driver and logistics coordinator, ensuring I arrived at physical therapy and class on time. She often enlisted help from family and friends to cover transportation when her schedule was tight. Part of her role was anticipating and addressing any obstacles that could disrupt our routine.

When I was still learning to use a wheelchair, the two of us did a dry run of the campus to scout out accessible entrances and find suitable parking. When we realized there were no parking options close to the building, she consulted campus police, who advised her to park out front while assisting me and to hang the disability placard from the rearview mirror.

The only time she refused to help me was when she got a parking ticket while parked outside the building, despite having the placard on full display. She sent me in alone to contest it, thinking that they wouldn't give a student using a wheelchair a hard time. I went in with the placard and the ticket, and she was right. They took care of it immediately.

My mother was also in charge of meals. Once we got our routine down, she stocked the fridge with healthy food that was easy to prepare when I was home alone during the day, along with everything I needed to pack lunches for campus. Our extended family also dropped off homemade meals to relieve some of the burden for my mother.

My brother took a different approach. He was less hands-on and more of a strategy guy. That worked out well, though, because he was living in Maryland at the time and was able to add value post-hospitalization from a distance. After I graduated from the walker to a four-pronged cane, I took a trip to visit him and my sister-in-law. One afternoon, he plopped down an issue of *U.S. News & World Report* on the table in front of me. It was the edition listing the top graduate schools. He told me, "Pick out a graduate school to go to, but I need the magazine back."

I followed his guidance and submitted applications to graduate schools to pursue research related to people with disabilities and assistive technology. In addition to being shaped by my own experiences, my mother's background in special education and assistive technology influenced my decision to pursue this route. I ended up going to graduate school, which was a pivotal step in preparing me for a career in social science research.

SUPPORT SERVICES AND THE PAPERWORK OLYMPICS

I couldn't ask for better support from my family. But navigating support services and the paperwork that came with it—that was a different story. That whole process felt like running a marathon, with an obstacle course thrown in for good measure. It required patience, persistence, and precision. I started by applying for Social Security disability benefits, but it turned out that the government didn't operate as quickly as my doctor, who offered me a disability parking tag on the spot.

I was denied the first time I applied, which wasn't a surprise. My mother knew someone who worked for Social Security, and she told us to expect that the first time around, so we appealed. Persistence and patience paid off, and it was determined that I met the eligibility criteria required to receive Social Security disability benefits. But without that insight through my mother's social connection, who knows if we would have appealed?

This experience amplifies the importance of being proactive in seeking out support services. When I started graduate school about two years later, I tapped into the university's Office for Students with Disabilities. They offered support depending on the accommodation that you needed. As someone with reduced mobility, I was eligible for paratransit services to get around campus, library assistance to retrieve books, periodicals, and other resources from the library stacks, and copy services (back then, hard copies were still all the rage).

I also applied for services from my state rehabilitation department. Once I was assessed and deemed eligible for these services, I was provided with equipment, including a laptop, training to help me learn how to drive again, and career services to support my job search after completing the graduate program.

By the time I started graduate school, which was about two years after having the surgery, the internet had become an essential part of academic life. The library services I received through the Office for Students with Disabilities were great, but having access to information at my fingertips without leaving my room was transformative, since getting around was still challenging. Plus, I had access to Kurzweil software, a text-to-speech program that was widely used by people with visual and learning disabilities back then. As an audio learner, the software made it much easier to keep up with my courses' discussion board posts and absorb course materials.

I learned how to drive again while in graduate school. For context, I was so excited to start driving when I was a teen, that I got my driver's license on my sixteenth birthday. But for me, relearning to drive after the surgery was terrifying.

At sixteen, there was no fear factor. The other cars on the road were like Barbie Dream Cars, harmless and almost toy-like. But as an adult who had not been behind the wheel in two years, every other car felt like a monster truck that was ready to flatten me.

I thought that learning to drive again would be like riding a bike. You just jump back in and get the hang of it. Instead, it felt more like doing your taxes—familiar, but still stressful. And with both, one mistake could have serious consequences.

Feeling intimidated by other vehicles was just part of the issue. I learned how to drive with no feeling in my right foot. Back then, the brake pedals of some vehicles were elevated enough from the floor that a foot could get stuck under them. I learned this firsthand when my mother let me try driving her minivan in an empty parking lot.

But there was a simple solution to my problem: Don't drive cars with an elevated brake pedal. I haven't encountered one of those in years. Still, whenever I rent a car, I practice moving my foot from the gas to the brake before turning on the ignition to make sure there are no gaps.

If my outcome had been reversed, with a weak right foot that I could feel, I'd likely need a car with hand controls. This would have meant learning to drive again would have involved more time, expense, and coordination. On top of this, renting a car with hand controls when traveling would have been an added logistical hurdle.

And if you're lingering on the fact that I'm driving without being able to feel my foot, don't worry. I had a full assessment with a rehab specialist who focuses on driving. The specialist assured me that the lack of sensation in my foot doesn't affect my ability to drive safely. But if we're ever together and my driving makes you nervous, I'm happy to kick back in the passenger seat. I'll bring my placard so we can score a great parking spot.

FROM SUPPORT SERVICES TO SOCIAL CIRCLES

For me, accessing disability support services wasn't just about getting help. It was also about finding community. During my first year of graduate school, I connected with the local Center for Independent Living. Not only did I learn about community resources, but I also built relationships with other people with and without disabilities who cared deeply about disability rights and community engagement. I began volunteer work doing administrative tasks at the Center, and later provided similar volunteer work for one of their clients. It turned out to be a good social outlet for me and gave me a greater sense of purpose.

This was a time in my life when I still felt limited by new

circumstances. But contributing to something bigger than myself helped shift my thinking from "all or nothing" to a more proactive mindset: even though I couldn't do *everything*, I could do *something*. That was the turning point when I stopped focusing on what I couldn't do and started embracing what I could.

• ● •

PERSON-CENTERED CARE DISCUSSION

Building a Support System

In this chapter, I've shared the ups and downs of building my support system—from leaning on family to tapping into social services. Looking back, some moments really showed what person-centered care can look like during the transition to community living. Others? Not so much. Here are a few examples of how my experiences lined up with the principles of person-centered care.

Alignment With Person-Centered Care

NAB Principle: Achieve Access to Meaningful Work and Activities

Access to meaningful work and activities means different things to different people. For me, the opportunity to attend graduate school was important and changed the course of my life. Given the uncertainty about my physical recovery, pursuing higher education was a strategic choice. It opened doors to meaningful work that didn't depend on physical strength. This path was made possible, in part, by the vocational guidance and support I received from my state rehabilitation agency.

Those services helped me build a professional foundation that included conducting research, delivering training, developing patient education materials, and even writing this book. The impact of vocational rehabilitation can be long-term and multidimensional, especially when it's delivered in a person-centered way.

While some may attach a stigma to receiving assistance from government-sponsored programs—or any type of help—I can say with confidence that I wouldn't have had many of my past work opportunities without that kind of support. And I'm not alone. National data show that in 2024, just 37.4% of people aged 16-64 with disabilities were employed, compared to 74.9% of those without disabilities.[1] For many, vocational rehabilitation can mean the difference between being sidelined and finding employment opportunities. A person-centered approach recognizes that individualized support—even beyond the clinical setting—can address social drivers of health and create lasting positive change.

Driving has also had a significant impact on my life, especially during a time when getting in cars with strangers just wasn't a thing. Instead of issuing a blanket "no," given the impaired sensation in my foot, a driving specialist took the time to apply the appropriate assessment criteria and guidelines, and I met the requirements to drive independently. This was a clear example of a solution tailored to the person, not just the condition. While not strictly medical, this service addressed a key social driver of health—transportation.

For me, developing the skills I needed to get work-ready and to drive in a region with limited public transportation was critical to putting the NAB principle of accessing meaningful work and activities into practice, and it remains essential to navigating life today.

But I also recognize that not everyone has access to the same level of support. Access to vocational rehabilitation services and adaptive driving assessments can vary depending on where a person lives, how well-resourced local programs are, and how visible or well-understood these services are within the community.

NAB Principle: Accelerate Access to Innovative Technologies

Keep in mind that in my early years of living with a disability, technology wasn't nearly as advanced as it is today. Back then, if someone had told me that wireless internet would be a thing, they might as well have added that teleportation would put the airline industry out of business. So, as I talk about "accelerating access to innovative technologies," remember that the tools I relied on in the late 1990s and early 2000s made a world of difference in making life easier back then.

One of technology's most powerful qualities is its adaptability. Tools originally designed for a specific purpose often end up benefiting a much broader audience. My physical condition made it difficult to access hard-copy materials. While library services offered some support, having online resources readily available transformed my sense of independence.

Similarly, mainstream features like voice recognition, text-to-speech, and word prediction, now standard on most mobile devices, were once primarily used within the disability community. While I didn't need text-to-speech software as a formal accommodation, it became an invaluable asset for my preferred learning style. This demonstrates how, when technology is designed to be accessible from the beginning, it empowers everyone, including people with disabilities, to choose the tools that best suit their unique needs. In fact, a 2024 article in *TechTrends* found that embedding accessibility and universal design into digital learning environments improved usability, engagement, and satisfaction for all users—not just those with disabilities.[2]

When technology is readily available, people can choose the supports that work best for them, fostering independence, participation, and inclusion. Ultimately, this can help accelerate opportunities for learning, work, and community engagement across the board. Prompt access to these innovations fosters independence, expands opportunities, and helps build a more inclusive society, aligning with the NAB's vision of accessible participation for all.

Opportunities for Person-Centered Care

NAB Principle: Ensure Full Access to Services and Supports

After transitioning home, accessing the broader network of services and supports, like disability benefits and vocational rehabilitation, felt like a drawn-out game of chicken, with each side waiting for the other to give up first. We were confronted with so many obstacles that it often felt as if the system was waiting for us to quit. But instead of blinking first, my parents drew on their professional know-how and personal networks to persevere.

That advantage, based on luck and circumstance, highlights a key reality: access to essential services and supports too often depends on one's ability to navigate complex systems and access to inside information. This creates an inequitable system where people without those resources face greater barriers to recovery and independence.

In fact, research shows that people with higher levels of social capital—like access to community organizations and supportive networks—have better health outcomes, while those with higher social vulnerability experience worse outcomes.[3] Not everyone has a family able to step in and advocate for them. That's why ensuring full access to services and supports is so vital. A systematic review found that interventions such as patient education, follow-up calls, and discharge planning significantly reduced hospital readmissions and emergency department visits. These findings demonstrate that well-structured care coordination during or immediately following hospital discharge is associated with smoother transitions and better outcomes.[4]

Person-centered care means ensuring that every individual can access support and services, regardless of their professional background, connections, or circumstances. When systems are easy to navigate and well-coordinated, patients and their families don't have to deal with bureaucracy and can focus on what matters most: their health and well-being.

NAB Principle: Value Dignity and Choice

The red tape surrounding disability insurance benefits didn't just wear down my patience—it took a toll on my self-esteem. After jumping through endless hoops just to apply for disability employment benefits, being denied felt like a personal blow. It made me question whether the physical pain, side effects from medication, and difficulty navigating my new body were all just figments of my imagination. *Maybe I was too soft and needed to tough it out*, I thought. In a way, the denial even made me feel guilty, like I was lazy and unworthy.

The principle of valuing dignity and choice is foundational to successful and sustainable long-term services and supports. Yet, my dignity was compromised at the very first barrier—accessing financial support through Social Security disability benefits, which can serve as a gateway to services like vocational rehabilitation, personal care, and community living.

While my experience was deeply uncomfortable, people facing more significant financial insecurity may encounter even greater layers of scrutiny and burden. One study found that low-income individuals seeking disability benefits were compelled to repeatedly "prove" their disability in ways that reinforced societal perceptions of them as the "unworthy poor," ultimately undermining their dignity, autonomy, and trust in the system.[5]

The true spirit of valuing dignity and choice applies to every interaction when accessing supports that make independent community living possible. Honoring this ideal affirms one's humanity and reinforces respect for those navigating difficult circumstances.

• • •

CONVERSATION STARTERS

Transitioning into community life with a disability reveals both the promises of person-centered care and the challenges when it is absent. Strong clinical, emotional, practical, and social support systems make all the difference. Consider the prompts below to reflect on how these dynamics have shaped your journey, your care, or your work.

For Patients, Providers, and Payers

Reflecting on the narrative in this chapter, are there additional moments where NAB principles were exemplified or fell short?

For Patients

1. Do you know how to check eligibility for local, state, or federal support programs for temporary or long-term support? These might include vocational rehabilitation, accessible transportation, or, for longer-term needs, Social Security disability benefits. If you're unsure what applies to your situation, who could you turn to for guidance—perhaps a caseworker, social worker, or advocacy organization?

2. When facing health concerns, what community resources, peer groups, online communities, or technologies could help you increase your independence or enhance your social life? Who could you reach out to for recommendations or support in connecting with these resources?

3. Whether you're battling the flu or recovering from a crisis, what daily tasks, such as meal prep, medication reminders, or errands, could you adapt in a way that spreads the effort without overwhelming anyone? What conversations might help clarify these roles and expectations?

4. How has technology helped you manage your health, access information, or maintain your independence? Are there new tools or features you could try to further support your goals?

For Providers

1. How do you stay current on community resources, peer groups, or technologies that address common social

drivers of health, such as transportation barriers, housing instability, or food insecurity?

2. How do you routinely screen for social drivers of health that could impact your patients' ability to follow care plans or attend appointments? What process do you have for connecting patients to appropriate resources or support services when these needs are identified?

3. When developing a care plan, do you ask patients about potential challenges in their daily lives, such as financial stress, work obligations, or caregiving responsibilities, that might affect their ability to manage their health? How does this information inform your recommendations or referrals?

4. How do you work with your care team to review insurance coverage and other benefit programs, ensuring that patients are not only aware of their options but also supported in overcoming access barriers related to cost, transportation, or health literacy?

For Payers

1. Do you offer policies with coverage that ensures prompt, affordable access to the full range of services, equipment, and therapies that support recovery and independent living? Do these policies keep pace with technological innovations that enhance accessibility, promote inclusion, and address social drivers of health?

2. How do you proactively identify and address financial, administrative, or systemic barriers, such as complex paperwork, prior authorizations, or narrow networks that can delay access to necessary care?

3. How do your policies uphold principles of person-centered care? For example, do they promote member dignity, autonomy, and choice? How might policies be updated to be more person-centered?

4. How are you addressing the emotional and psychological needs of members experiencing significant physical changes, such as connecting them to counseling, peer support, or social networks?

SEVEN

FINDING YOUR SWEET SPOT

RESEARCH, MEDS, AND GETTING
YOUR DOCTOR TO SWIPE RIGHT

I wish I could offer a roadmap to help navigate patients' next steps, but everyone's journey is different. What works for one person may not work for another. For me, it has always been about balancing expert medical advice with a willingness to explore different treatment options—sometimes even those that weren't covered in medical school (but with my doctor's blessing).

It's important to recognize that not all information is created equal, especially when it comes to health. Whether considering prescription medications or natural remedies, I prioritize sources grounded in science, reviewed by experts, and transparent about their limitations. I believe this is the "responsible" approach (yes, those are air quotes with a side of eye rolling), but let's be real—it's not always the approach that feels good. Change is hard, and sometimes the facts can be a tough pill to swallow—literally and figuratively.

Take my cholesterol and Hemoglobin A1c (which is like a three-month report card for blood sugar), for example. When both were outside the recommended range, I knew I needed to turn things around because I didn't want to go on medication. My doctor suggested seeing a registered dietitian, but I insisted I could change my diet on my own. Well, time went by, and nothing changed. I eventually came to terms with the harsh reality that I needed backup, and I agreed to see a dietitian.

Even though it was my choice to see the dietitian, I was a bit defiant at our first appointment. When she asked what brought me in, I told her, "A court order." I was joking—sort of. Truth is, I was frustrated. After being a vegetarian for more than three decades, I figured I'd have my nutrition all figured out, but I still didn't have the know-how to control my cholesterol on my own.

Despite my initial resistance, working with the dietitian turned out to be a really positive experience. She reviewed my medical history to tailor her recommendations for safety and effectiveness. I committed to making changes, like eating more balanced meals and having smaller portions more frequently throughout the day. And you know what? My cholesterol levels improved significantly after making these modifications to my diet and eating habits.

When it came to the grade on my blood sugar report card, it was a different story. I expected to see some movement after all my efforts. But that number didn't budge. (Turns out, eating more frequently throughout the day doesn't include extra desserts.) It was frustrating, but sometimes even our best efforts don't immediately show up in the numbers. I wish good health could happen on autopilot, but it really comes down to persistence and close collaboration with trusted medical professionals.

Whenever I've explored options that didn't involve my doctor as a matchmaker—like acupuncture for pain management—I've still made sure to discuss them during appointments. Personally, I would never pursue anything my medical professional advises against. This helps me steer clear of misinformation and helps me make decisions rooted in the best available knowledge, not just hope or hype. At the same time, I know the world is much bigger than a doctor's office. I spend most of my life outside those four walls and want to keep searching for solutions—again, with my doctor's blessing.

That's why I'm open to seeking second opinions. In fact, second opinions can lead to a different diagnosis in complex cases and may change your care plan and even your life.[1] I'm also open to exploring natural remedies. For example, I've added ginger to my diet for its anti-inflammatory properties (plus, it tastes really good). But I also recognize that "natural" doesn't always mean risk-free, as ginger, for instance, can interact with blood thinners. Plus, sometimes natural remedies just aren't enough. Like when the incision from my spinal cord surgery became infected, I needed more than essential oils and a deep tissue massage—I needed *serious* muscle: antibiotics.

I offer these examples to demonstrate how the expertise of medical professionals has been critical to my recovery, and so has exploring options. Listening to medical science doesn't mean patients should remain silent.

With all those caveats, here's how I found my "sweet spot" when it came to managing my health. Again, I'm just sharing my own experience—it's important that you discuss your approach to healthcare with your medical professional.

SOMETIMES, MEDICINE IS A DOUBLE-EDGED SWORD

I'm open to taking prescription medication when it's medically necessary, like when my bone density was low and I ended up with a fractured toe. In situations like that, I'll take what's prescribed.

However, my attitude shifts when it comes to medicine for chronic pain and discomfort. I tend to weigh the pros and cons much more carefully. For example, I was prescribed two medications for spasticity, but I really disliked the side effects. One of them is known to have a risk of dependence or addiction, which made me uneasy. I was told to take it "as needed," so I reserved it for only the worst flare-ups.

The other medication was meant to be taken regularly. Not only did I hate how it made me feel, but I also questioned whether I wanted to be on it long-term. Sure, the risk of liver damage was said to be small, but I didn't want to find out decades later that I'd become one of the rare cases. That's when I made a really bad decision: I stopped taking it on my own. It led to agitation and insomnia, but I was determined and managed to quit cold turkey. I share this as a cautionary tale, not as a suggestion.

Later, during a conversation with a friend who's a doctor, I learned that quitting that particular medication abruptly can actually trigger seizures and hallucinations in some cases. That's when I realized how important it is to modify medications only under medical supervision—even when you're eager to be done with them.

Looking back, I realize that no one ever asked if I was still taking my prescription during follow-up appointments, and I never brought it up myself. Turns out, "don't ask, don't tell" isn't the best approach in healthcare. This whole situation underscores the importance of consulting your doctor before making changes to prescribed medications and being proactive about sharing information. Now, even if doctors don't ask, I still make sure to tell.

Years after my spinal cord surgery, the FDA approved a drug for neuropathic pain in people with spinal cord injuries that was originally developed for a different purpose. I did a little digging and found that this particular class of drugs increased the risk of suicidal thoughts. Even though the likelihood of this happening was low, for me, that risk was a deal breaker since it wasn't medically necessary.

Fast forward a year or so, I was sitting next to a man on an airplane who told me that his wife had been prescribed that medication and, personality-wise, had turned into a different person after taking it. This conversation made me grateful that I did not pursue that option. I'm not saying others shouldn't consider it, but for me, it's important to weigh the trade-offs and make decisions based on my priorities and risk tolerance.

JUST WHAT THE DOCTOR ORDERED?

I've learned that when it comes to medication, the "why" matters just as much as the "what." So whenever a doctor suggests a new prescription, I try to get clear on what it's supposed to do—whether it's solving a health problem, managing symptoms, or simply making me more comfortable. That clarity shapes how I weigh the risks, side effects, and alternatives. Part of this mindset goes back to when I was experiencing pain from the hemorrhaged AVM and taking medicine that silenced some very important messages my body was trying to tell me. Now, I've learned to pause and consider what the pain itself might mean.

If it's for symptom relief, I consider whether the symptom is actually a warning sign and ask my doctor what it would mean if the medication just masks the problem. I also wonder about side effects that could lead to other health issues or interfere with my ability to work or engage in other activities that are important to me. Finally, I consider alternatives that may be available, like a lifestyle change or even a different type of medication if I have concerns about the original suggestion.

When I try a new medicine, I read labels carefully to double- and triple-check things like warnings and dosage amounts. Pharmacists are human, and on more than one occasion, I've been given medications that didn't match what the doctor prescribed. Though I'm not a medical expert, I try to do what is in my control to make sure that medicine is working for me and not against me.

Medication instructions can sometimes be a bit confusing. Take "do not take with alcohol," for example. Does that mean you should abstain completely while on the medicine, or just don't take your prescription pills with a glass of wine? As written, that warning hits differently with your morning cereal than it does at happy hour. If the instructions are open to interpretation, it's important to ask a pharmacist for clarification before making a decision that could have negative health consequences. Even if you get your medications by mail order, you can still empower yourself with information by calling the pharmacist to ask questions or request a consultation.

UNLOCKING THE MYSTERIES OF YOUR PERMANENT RECORD

One of the most overlooked and important things I've done to support my care is staying on top of what's in my medical chart. Remember how teachers used to warn us about our "permanent record"? Turns out, your real one lives at your doctor's office. Whatever your provider writes becomes part of your health history, and other providers will rely on it to make decisions about your future care.

You probably never asked to see your records back in school, but now? Go for it. Reviewing your doctor's notes helps ensure they capture what matters, and gives you a chance to provide clarity.

Take the abbreviation "WNL," for example—it stands for "within normal limits." Sounds reassuring, right? And maybe it is. But sometimes it shows up even when a test wasn't done, thanks to copy-paste habits or auto-filled templates in electronic health records. "Normal" results might get logged without anyone ever checking you.[2]

Even when a test *is* performed, "normal" isn't always one-size-fits-all. The data behind those limits often comes from studies that don't reflect the full population. If you don't match the demographics used in the research—like race, ethnicity, sex, or age—those "normal" ranges might not apply to you.

For example, research shows that creatinine levels can differ across populations. Healthy people of Asian descent, for instance, may have lower average levels than what some U.S. lab ranges consider "within normal limits." Without context, a perfectly healthy result could get flagged as abnormal. That can lead to unnecessary tests, extra costs, and a whole lot of worry for no good reason.[3] This amplifies why "normal" isn't always universal. It also demonstrates how differences in populations, if not accounted for carefully, can contribute to disparities in care.

Emergency situations can pose real challenges to documentation, and there may not always be time to capture every detail in the moment. But once the immediate crisis passes, accurate records support safety, continuity of care, and peace of mind.

Bottom line: you and your providers are partners. You have valuable insight to contribute. And it's totally reasonable to review your medical record the same way you'd review the check after a meal, just to make sure everything adds up.

RELIEF REROUTED

Even after hospital discharge, I struggled, struggled, struggled with constipation. I was so desperate for help that I'd talk to anyone about it. My healthcare providers recommended enemas, suppositories, stool softeners, and oral medications, but these weren't long-term solutions for me. Who wants to rely on something for the rest of their life just to not feel bloated?

My own research, coupled with trial and error, led me to options that provided me relief, like drinking tons of water, eating leafy greens, adding ground flaxseed, and trying MSM (a naturally occurring compound). These weren't originally part of my doctors' recommendations, but I brought them up during appointments and made sure they wouldn't interfere with my treatment. I share this not as a suggestion, but as an invitation to explore additional options you can discuss with your healthcare provider. That step is important because even something considered "natural" might not interact well with other parts of your treatment plan.

I had a similar situation with pain. Lower back aches and neuropathic pain in my legs were constant companions after my surgery. Sometimes, I could distract myself from the pain, but it was always there. For my lower back aches, a chance conversation with a presenter at a conference led me to try acupuncture. I was skeptical, but after doing my homework, I gave it a shot. To my surprise, it worked. Effectiveness varies for different people and conditions, but it made my lower back aches vanish. Unfortunately, acupuncture didn't put a dent in the neuropathic pain that I experience to this day, but I still keep looking for solutions.

WATCH OUT FOR WILD ASSUMPTIONS

Assumptions in healthcare settings can shape patient-provider relationships and impact care. Factual information is the foundation of trust and shared decision-making. Patients play a key role by offering their providers all the details needed to make the best recommendations, while providers have a responsibility to seek facts and not rely on assumptions.

I learned this firsthand in graduate school when I had a quick trip to the hospital after an episode of dizziness, lightheadedness, and fatigue. When the attending physician was examining me, she asked what I did for a living. I told her I was a doctoral student. She immediately asked if I was a doctoral student at a nearby regional university. When her question was met with silence, she followed up with, "Or here at 'The U'?"

For context, I was a doctoral student at the university affiliated with the hospital where I was receiving treatment. This prestigious Big Ten research university is internationally recognized for its academic rigor. The hospital is part of the same healthcare system that provided my primary care, and I used health insurance administered through this institution.

The university she assumed I was attending is a respected regional public university located in the same county and known for its commitment to community engagement, a supportive learning environment, and student success.

Given my setting and circumstances, her first assumption stood out to me. That moment made me wonder what led her to that conclusion—was it something about how I looked, spoke, or presented myself? It also left me reflecting on what other unspoken assumptions might be shaping our interaction.

Even highly trained professionals are human, and we all carry mental shortcuts that may not match reality. In everyday life, these assumptions can be awkward or uncomfortable. But in healthcare, they can have real consequences for diagnosis, treatment, and how patients are perceived and supported.

This experience reinforced the importance of being explicit and thorough when communicating with providers. As patients, we sometimes need to "hand-feed" information to ensure our story is understood. For providers, it's a reminder that while it's hard to control assumptions, you can choose not to act on them. Instead, respect your patients' voices and listen to the facts.

WAIT, THE THERAPIST DOES THE WORK?

I am confident that I received the best care available in 1997. My surgeon was ahead of his time, but science and technology have advanced since then. Today, there are new medications, improved rehab tools, and different methodologies that simply didn't exist back then. I've tried some of the newer medications to ease my leg discomfort, but none have impressed me. What did make a difference was returning to physical therapy.

I started off at a boutique private practice called Elite Physical Therapy for orthopedic physical therapy, which focused on strengthening my muscles and improving my flexibility to help me move better and reduce pain. If you like working out, you'd love going to orthopedic physical therapy. If you don't like working out, you'd love leaving orthopedic physical therapy. I fell clearly in that second group, except for the days when my therapist did manual therapy. Who knew physical therapy could involve the therapist doing all the work?

On some days, during the last ten minutes of the session, she'd take me to a private treatment room and manually stretch out my muscles. Yes, it had medical benefits, but it felt so good that I'm sure she used it as a secret weapon to keep me coming back.

My therapist also did dry needling with electrical stimulation, which combined needles and gentle electrical currents to release tension when my muscles were extra tight. It reminded me of acupuncture, but with bigger needles and electricity. This may sound like more of an interrogation technique than a treatment, but I actually thought it felt pretty good. I just made sure to leave my bottled water at the door. Jokes aside, I'm actually terrified of needles, but I found dry needling with electrical stimulation to be so effective (and even comfortable) that I have recommended it to others.

Once I completed my orthopedic physical therapy, my therapist explored opportunities for me to transition into neurological (or neuro) rehabilitation. Neuro-rehab is designed for people with injuries or disorders impacting the nervous system, including the brain and spinal cord. Learning how to walk again isn't like one of those babies in a Huggies commercial that just finds its footing and dashes away. It's taken structured retraining after my surgery, and the need for additional retraining between the brain and the muscles has remained over the years (admittedly, I need to act on that more than I do).

Focused re-education offered through neuro-rehab helps improve muscle coordination and my walking pattern, or gait. It's sort of like couples counseling for your brain and your muscles— sometimes they need a therapist to work through their issues.

My orthopedic therapist ended up referring me to the Kennedy Krieger Institute for neurological rehabilitation. This huge facility is known for its interdisciplinary team approach, use of state-of-the-art equipment, and innovative therapies backed by groundbreaking research. At first, I was on the fence about going because I didn't want to drive the thirty-five minutes it takes to get there. But I got on board when I found out it was a destination facility that drew people from all over the country. It's like Disney, but instead of standing in long lines to get on rides, everyone gets a "fast pass" to use all of the equipment.

At the Kennedy Krieger Institute, I was treated by an amazing team that consisted of a physical therapist, a physician, and a nurse. I benefited from equipment and techniques I hadn't experienced in earlier years.

Medical advancements have come a long way since having spinal cord surgery all those years ago. Today, less-invasive proce-dures and more targeted treatments might have led to a smoother recovery—or even a different outcome altogether. While I can't go back in time armed with modern medicine for a do-over (at least not until modern science surprises us with a time machine), I'm grateful there are opportunities to benefit from ongoing progress in medical science and rehabilitation.

• • •

PERSON-CENTERED CARE DISCUSSION

Exploring Healthcare Options

The ongoing search for optimal health outcomes is filled with hits and misses. Here's a look at where my experiences tracked with person-centered care—and where they didn't quite land.

Alignment With Person-Centered Care

NAB Principle: Improve Health and Well-being Through Individual Empowerment and System Coordination

My experience returning to physical therapy demonstrates how systems coordination can improve health and well-being. Even though I had no clue about the difference between orthopedic and neurological physical therapy, the orthopedic therapist did. When she took me as far as possible, she didn't just send me on my way. She empowered me with the information and tools to keep moving forward by connecting me to the neuro-rehab facility. As a bonus, I had the benefit of a multidisciplinary team working together to figure out what I needed next.

An interdisciplinary teamwork approach involving physical therapists, physicians, and nurses closely collaborating can help overcome organizational and professional barriers, and tailored strategies can further support this approach.[4] This is the NAB principle in action—healthcare systems working in sync to coordinate care while empowering patients with the knowledge, support, and agency needed to actively shape their path forward.

NAB Principle: Value Dignity and Choice

One size rarely fits all, not just with long-term support services, but also in healthcare and rehabilitation. The best care occurs when it's flexible and collaborative, tailored to the individual rather than forcing the individual to fit into a rigid system. But this can only work when a patient's dignity, personal strengths, and right to self-determination are truly valued.

For example, my doctors didn't suggest acupuncture, but they didn't dismiss it either. They recognized it was safe to try and gave me the freedom to explore a treatment that suited my needs. This experience aligns with a 2023 scoping review, which highlights that flexible, individualized care plans incorporating patient input are a key component of integrated care models, particularly for chronic and complex conditions.[5]

Valuing dignity and choice doesn't mean that healthcare providers step back or stop guiding their patients. Instead, it means building real partnerships, offering options, listening carefully, and asking questions like "What matters most to you about your health?" "How does this affect your life, both now and in the future?" and "Are there other concerns you'd like us to consider?"

When providers engage with patients in this way, they build trust and help people gain the skills and confidence to take charge of their own care. Ultimately, honoring dignity, personal strengths, and self-determination leads to better outcomes and a more positive, empowering healthcare experience for everyone.

Opportunities for Person-Centered Care

Achieving Community Inclusion and Full Participation

This NAB principle supports the need for people not just to exist in the world, but to fully participate in everyday life. Engagement goes beyond physical access; it includes respectful social interaction. People need to be acknowledged, heard, and treated with dignity.

When I went to the hospital as a graduate student, the doctor's assumption about where I attended school caught me off guard. She made that assumption not based on anything I said, but on how she perceived me.

Experiences like this go beyond personal discomfort. They can impact a person's ability to fully engage in their healthcare. Misjudging or dismissing patients in healthcare settings can erode trust and discourage participation in care decisions. Research indicates that assumptions based on appearance or background can contribute to diagnostic errors and interfere with appropriate care.[6]

True person-centered care means seeking accurate information through active listening rather than relying on assumptions. This helps create environments where patients feel safe, respected, and like they belong. It's especially critical when patients come from different cultural backgrounds or identities than their providers, as the risk of misunderstandings or knowledge gaps increases. While emergency situations often require swift decisions, taking time to check assumptions and preserve a patient's dignity is key to building trust and encouraging meaningful engagement in their care.

NAB Principle: Ensure Full Access to Services and Supports

Even though I've benefited from great medical care, there was still room for more support from my medical team. Perhaps most concerning was the lack of guidance about what could happen if I stopped taking a prescribed medication. In fairness, the warnings were probably stated clearly in 0.5 font on the medicine bottle. But small print aside, the reality is that deviating from prescribed medication instructions is actually pretty common.

In fact, studies have highlighted that medication nonadherence is a common challenge for many patients.[7] Given this trend, patients would benefit from more targeted support around medication management, particularly those managing multiple prescriptions, including many older adults and people with disabilities.

This ordeal demonstrates that access goes beyond getting a prescription to include a full range of supports needed to use treatments safely and maintain independence. Medications—especially those with serious health risks—require conversations, planning, and follow-up. Aligning care with this principle means ensuring that people have both access to medication and the information they need to make medicine meaningful and safe.

• • •

CONVERSATION STARTERS

When you're ill, in pain, or uncomfortable, it can feel like you'll do anything for relief. How are you ensuring that your safety—or the safety of patients or members—is being protected throughout that process? The discussion questions below are meant to help spark discussions and reflection.

For Patients, Providers, and Payers

Reflecting on the narrative in this chapter, are there additional moments where NAB principles were exemplified or fell short?

For Patients

1. When you think about your last medical appointment, what steps did you take ahead of time to make sure you understood the information and got your key questions

answered? What made you feel prepared—or what do you wish you'd done differently to feel more confident, engaged, or in control during the visit?

2. If you're interested in trying complementary therapies, such as changing your diet, acupuncture, or supplements, or exploring new medical techniques, how can you safely consider these options and discuss them with your care team to make sure they won't interfere with your current treatments or cause harm?

3. What strategies can help you communicate with your healthcare provider if you feel unsure or have concerns about a treatment, medication, or recommendation?

4. How can you advocate for yourself if you sense a healthcare provider is making assumptions about your background, needs, or goals instead of truly listening to you? What practical strategies, questions, or supports might help you feel empowered to speak up to foster a truly collaborative approach to your care, even in situations where it might feel uncomfortable or intimidating to question the doctor?

For Providers

1. Recognizing that many clinicians receive limited formal education in complementary therapies, how do you stay informed and guide patients who inquire about alternative or integrative treatments? How do you decide when to seek input from specialists or refer patients to trusted resources?

2. How do you recognize and address potential gaps in truly understanding your patients, especially when

considering factors such as language differences, health literacy, cultural beliefs, or religious practices? What strategies do you use to ensure you're actively listening and not making assumptions about their backgrounds, needs, or goals, and how do you seek understanding when needed?

3. How do you support patients in advocating for themselves, and what resources do you provide to help them become active partners in their care?

4. Is there a time when a patient's feedback or advocacy led you to change your approach to care? What did you learn from that experience?

For Payers

1. How do you engage members in decisions about their care when requirements like prior authorization may impact treatment options, especially if therapies are outside of standard clinical protocols or in emerging areas?

2. How do you determine which alternative or complementary therapies, such as acupuncture, chiropractic care, or nutritional therapies, are covered under your healthcare plans, and what steps do you take to help patients understand their coverage options and support them if their preferred approach is not included?

3. What resources or support do you provide to help members navigate complex coverage issues and advocate for themselves when they have questions or concerns about their benefits?

4. What specific initiatives help members stay on track with their prescribed care, avoid risky discontinuations or harmful interactions, and encourage questions about medication safety, especially for those managing multiple conditions or considering complementary therapies? How do you use feedback to improve quality and person-centered support system-wide?

"Hey, you don't fall... how you gonna know what gettin' up is like?"
–Attributed to Bernard ("B. Nard"), Roll Bounce (2005)

PART C: STRUTTING WITH SWAG

THE (NOT SO) FINE PRINT ABOUT PART C

Parts A and B covered my journey from hospitals back into the community, which was a mix of challenges, support, and good fortune. But adapting and searching for answers didn't end there. It continues to evolve throughout my life.

In Part C, Strutting with Swag, I invite you into my world today. My life is rich and fulfilling, yet undeniably marked by the effects of the arteriovenous malformation in my spinal cord, the care I received to address it, and even the bewilderment at the cost of healthcare in the United States. Nevertheless, the experiences I had during recovery opened doors to education and professional opportunities I might never have pursued otherwise.

This section takes a different approach from earlier parts. Rather than presenting frameworks and guiding questions, I share lessons I continue to learn today as I pursue wellness, manage my health, and navigate life with a disability.

Chapters 8-9 Explore:

- Living with disability, navigating independence, and ongoing wellness through real-world strategies and reflections.
- Financial and policy considerations that impact person-centered care.

After Chapter 9, I acknowledge barriers that can keep person-centered care from becoming standard practice, and provide actionable strategies to help patients, providers, and payers make it a reality. I close with heartfelt "love letters" to each of these three groups.

EIGHT

I'M STILL STANDING

(WITH ELTON PLAYING AND A CHAIR STANDING BY)

When I was first diagnosed all those years ago, I was scared that I was going to die. Once I realized I would live, but would likely go through life with a disability, I faced other types of fears. I worried about what people would think of me. Would their perceptions limit my opportunities, shape my future, or even define who I was?

Back then, I would have given anything to know how my life was going to turn out. I think the problem was that, in my mind, I gave too much power to my fears. I let them influence how I saw my future and how I saw myself. I thought being disabled meant my life wouldn't be great because of those fears.

Over time, I realized that I had far more power to guide my destiny than my fears did. Sure, people would think what they wanted and might even treat me differently. It might not feel good, and it might not even be fair, but the less time I spent worrying about what other people thought, the more time I had to focus on things that truly mattered to me—and the more power I had to direct my future.

Here's a snapshot of where things stand today. Since we've already mapped person-centered care to my earlier experiences, I now focus on different parts of my life to show how these values show up, both in my doctor's office and everywhere else I go.

STILL STANDING, BUT BRING ME A CHAIR: MY BODY TODAY

When I first had spinal cord surgery, I was so curious about how my recovery would turn out. Fast forward all of these years, and I'm feeling great! I still walk with a limp, and my balance could be better, which means I get to use a very cool clear cane to get around. Some people think it's just a prop or a fashion statement, but the only statement it's making is "Where's the elevator?"

The hardest part of my physical condition isn't how I move; it's the neuropathic pain that I experience every minute of every day. I feel it under my skin.

The best way I can describe it? That nine-volt battery test some of us did as kids—touching the metal circles to your tongue to see if it had juice. If you felt a shock, it did. If not, it was drained.

The good news: most of the batteries I tested had power.

The bad news: most of the batteries I tested had power.

Ever since the surgery, my right foot and leg have felt a milder version of that "battery-on-the-tongue" pain, twenty-four hours a day, seven days a week. Given the choice, I would absolutely choose the limp over that pain.

And here's what's wild. At the surface level, I have no feeling in much of my right foot and leg. I don't notice injuries like cuts or burns until I see blood, skin discoloration, or swelling. My right leg always feels like it's wearing a corset—just without the slimming effect.

Over the years, I've come to adapt to this discomfort and to a world that isn't built for people with disabilities. But I welcome new insights that help me live better—even in small ways.

Recently, during a routine doctor's appointment, I mentioned to my primary care physician that my legs hurt more on days when I stay home and don't move around much. She told me that movement was important for pain management, something I had definitely observed but never knew was a medical fact.

That conversation reinforced for me that there's always something new to discover, and it reminded me of the importance of being open to learning new things. It also demonstrates what good care looks like—collaborative, curious, and centered on my lived experience. That's person-centered care in action: a doctor who listens, considers what I've noticed about my own body, and builds on it.

One unexpected result of dealing with mobility issues is that I've become a master of efficiency. I'm always scanning for the shortest route, the smoothest surface, or the easiest way to get from point A to point B. When steps take a lot of effort, you start seeing every situation as a game to be solved in the fewest moves possible. This mindset has spilled over into other areas of my life, making me a champion shortcut-finder and a big fan of anything that saves time or energy.

LOOKING BACK, MOVING FORWARD: THOUGHTS ON THE PAST AND FUTURE

While I've gotten better at navigating the day-to-day, every now and then, I look back and wonder, what if things had gone differently? Don't get me wrong; I'm at peace with how things turned out. But "what if" moments still surface now and then, especially when I think about the advancements in medicine since my spinal cord surgery in 1997.

Back then, I received the best care available, which meant a highly manual approach: opening my spine and operating directly inside the spinal cord to remove the AVM. It was risky and complicated. Today, surgical approaches have evolved to sometimes be less invasive. Advances in technology and surgical precision have lowered some risks and improved recovery times. Sometimes, I wonder whether, with today's tools and options, I might have made a fuller recovery.

Recently, about twenty-five years after my surgery, I had a new MRI to see how things have changed. When I brought my original films from 1997 for comparison, the radiology team couldn't read them because their equipment was incompatible with the old film format. The shift from film to digital imaging means that older records may become inaccessible as technology advances. This disconnect made it difficult to directly compare my past and present images, demonstrating how progress in technology can sometimes create new barriers for long-term care.

Although medical techniques have advanced rapidly, the approach to engaging patients hasn't kept pace. Dr. Epstein was a pioneer in developing new treatments for spinal cord conditions, and science has since built on his methodologies. However, his ability to balance medical expertise with a holistic, person-centered approach remains novel in many healthcare settings, even today. Despite growing recognition that involving patients as active partners leads to better outcomes, true patient partnership still lags behind the rapid advances in medical science and technology.

This gap isn't simply a matter of will. Many providers face intense pressure from high patient volumes, administrative burdens, and limited time, which makes engaging in deeper conversations more difficult. These constraints can hinder the moments of patient-provider connection that are essential for person-centered care.

LOW-TECH HACKS, HIGH-TECH HELP: STRATEGIES THAT PERSONALIZE MY WELL-BEING

I wish I could snap my fingers and make the world more accessible. Since I can't, I focus on what I *can* control—how I care for myself and adapt to daily life. I'm always thinking up life hacks to make my environment work better for me.

Many of my strategies are simple, like using a magnet to pick up bobby pins from the floor—a hack I learned from my first MRI experience. When emptying the dishwasher, I use a dishpan to transport a pile of dishes at once so I don't have to walk back and forth from the dishwasher to the cupboards. I also choose baths when I'm at home over showers.

Sure, baths are relaxing and make my legs feel good, but it's also much harder to fall when you're already sitting down. Shower chairs are an option, too, but I've never been a big fan. These are just a few small steps that make a big difference in my daily life.

Physical activity can be challenging, but it's a cornerstone of my self-care. I love the idea of being fit; I just wish it didn't take so much motivation. That's why I gravitate toward technology that, for me, makes things easier and more practical.

One of my best discoveries has been the Supernatural app, a virtual reality (VR) fitness platform I use on my VR headset. It features a team of virtual coaches who are personable and encouraging. They guide me through squats and arm movements as I strike balloons with a bat, while some of my favorite music plays through the headset. Plus, the scenery transports me to places like South

Africa, Greece, and Switzerland, all from the comfort of my living room.

The app also includes modifiers for different disabilities. I turn off the knee-strike feature because of my balance, but users can also disable squats, switch to a forward-facing mode (great for athletes who use wheelchairs), or even play with just one controller if needed.

I know virtual reality exercise isn't for everyone. But the best workout is the one I actually do, not just the one I think about doing while binge-watching *The Amazing Race*. For me, virtual reality has been a surprisingly great option.

Technology has made managing my health so much easier. Health insurance apps are helpful for tracking records, but my One Medical subscription has truly been a game-changer. One Medical is a primary care practice that also offers a membership that provides 24/7 access to on-demand virtual care services. The One Medical app streamlines my healthcare—organizing records, tracking next steps, communicating with providers, and scheduling appointments. If I need to see a specialist, One Medical coordinates referrals directly with healthcare systems and stores everything I need in the app, making access to care seamless.

My primary care physician (whom I love) addresses both routine and chronic health needs, listens attentively, and works with me to find solutions that feel right for both of us. It's the closest thing to enjoyable healthcare I can imagine—and when I actually enjoy something, I'm much more likely to stick with it.

One Medical has fit so seamlessly into my life that it even travels with me. I've used it to get blood work done across the country during a free hour before hotel check-in and accessed care for urgent needs in other cities.

Once, when I developed a skin abscess right before a trip, I booked a virtual appointment hours before I was scheduled to fly out. The One Medical physician told me I needed to be seen in person. When I explained that I had a flight to catch, she found a One Medical doctor along my route to the airport, booked the appointment, and sent in a prescription for antibiotics.

Even though she wasn't my regular doctor, all of my records, including pharmacy information, were linked to my profile. I picked up my prescription, swung by the appointment (with a one-block detour from my route), got examined, and received care instructions. The doctor even scheduled a follow-up at a One Medical near home. After all of that, I still made my flight. This is healthcare designed around me, not just my diagnosis—exactly the kind of integration and ease that person-centered care strives for.

Here's what One Medical reminds me of—though they might not appreciate the comparison. It's got the customization of Burger King, the courtesy of Chick-fil-A, and the nostalgic charm of McDonald's. It's healthcare where I actually get what I want, I'm treated kindly, and I even look forward to showing up. (Now, if I could only get them to serve fries in the waiting room, I'd know they took my feedback seriously.)

While technology, like virtual reality fitness and streamlined healthcare apps, has made managing my health more personal and manageable, I'm also keenly aware of the rapidly evolving role of artificial intelligence (AI) in healthcare. AI offers interesting possibilities to further customize care to individual needs, but also presents new challenges and uncertainties that are worth exploring. For instance, during a 2024 mammogram, I was offered an AI-powered analysis to help radiologists detect subtle signs of cancer. I opted in and paid out of pocket for this add-on, believing early detection improves outcomes.

I felt cautiously optimistic about my choice, but it's important to remember that AI in healthcare is still in its early stages. Some studies suggest AI can help radiologists improve breast cancer detection, yet researchers caution that many tools are trained on limited data sets, potentially reducing effectiveness across diverse populations. Researchers emphasize the need for more large-scale trials and greater transparency to ensure AI is safe, equitable, and reliable in everyday care.[1]

Health insurers typically require strong evidence that a tool improves real-world outcomes before considering reimbursement. This means more large-scale clinical trials and validation studies demonstrating effectiveness and value are needed before AI-based services like the one I chose become routinely covered.[2]

In many ways, AI is a double-edged sword in healthcare. While it holds great promise to personalize treatment, it also raises serious concerns—such as lack of transparency in decision-making, potential algorithmic bias, and data privacy issues. These concerns have been voiced by both the public and healthcare professionals.[3]

AI may also affect the patient-provider relationship. One study found that doctors who disclose their use of AI are perceived as less competent, trustworthy, and empathetic than those who do not, leading patients to be less willing to book appointments with them.[4] While transparency is essential, this underscores the need to clearly demonstrate how AI is used responsibly for the benefit of patients to build trust and strengthen patient-provider partnerships.

STRANGERS ASSUME, FRIENDS FORGIVE: THE TRUTH BEHIND THE CANE

I think it's great that offerings like Supernatural and One Medical recognize that different users have different needs. I just wish that more of the assumptions people make about disabilities were as thoughtful and productive. Instead, I sometimes encounter lower expectations or a level of sympathy I might not otherwise receive. It almost feels like I'm seen as just a diagnosis or stereotype, rather than a whole person (which includes having a disability).

There's also a constant stream of unsolicited advice: how to walk, what to try, what might "fix" me. Again, all offered in the spirit of trying to be helpful. But if you think backseat drivers are bad, try living half your life with backseat walkers. Strangers sometimes stop me on the street to pray that I'll walk straight (can I get a witness, 'cause I know I'm not alone). I try to appreciate the positive intention behind such comments, but I wish people didn't see me as someone who needs to be fixed. I feel great about my life and who I am. This is my reality, and I'm content with it.

Friends and close acquaintances are a different story. I actually *want* them to know about that part of my life. I'm surprised—and even feel a bit guilty—when I realize that someone important to me doesn't know the backstory behind my disability. And that's because it's such an important part of my life. It's one of many things that make Cynthia, Cynthia. That's on me—it's not something I try to keep private. I just don't think about it enough to bring it up in conversation. But that's my take. Not everyone shares my position.

Most people in my inner circle are probably too polite to ask, even if they're curious. And, of course, some people simply don't care, which is totally fine. One of the trends I've noticed among my inner circle is that, when they sense I might need help, their response is based on what's actually happening in the moment—not on assumptions from a quick glance—and they respond by asking, listening, and responding to what I truly need. It's almost like they have inside knowledge of a certain healthcare model, whether they know it or not (wink, wink).

HOW DISABILITY LED TO DEGREES OF OPPORTUNITY

Even though my spinal cord injury brought new challenges, it also set my life on a path I might never have otherwise considered. I went on to earn two master's degrees and a doctorate, which proved invaluable since my stamina isn't suited for jobs that require a lot of physical activity. Graduate school provided me with the opportunity to develop skills that enabled me to rely more on my mind than my body in my career.

My advanced degrees in technology and disability opened doors to projects that expanded access to innovative technology for people with disabilities, advanced disability policy, and led to opportunities to serve on various advisory committees focused on improving outcomes for people with disabilities. At the same time, my master's in communications strengthened my work in knowledge translation, helping me to distill dense medical research into practical, user-friendly information for those who need it to improve their health and social outcomes.

The phrase "social drivers of health" wasn't always in my vocabulary. But looking back, I see how my educational experience led to professional opportunities that play to my strengths. My career helped build the confidence and analytical skills I've relied on to advocate for my care. I used to think of education and career milestones as just markers of success. In reality, they're powerful social drivers that spark curiosity, sharpen self-advocacy, and open doors to actively participate in person-centered care. Yet healthcare should be accessible to everyone, regardless of education or social circumstances.

ACTIVATING THAT "CAN-DO" SPIRIT

As much potential as there is in our healthcare system, I've learned that lasting change takes time. In the meantime, I've had to make the most of what's within my control—whether that means navigating the system's hurdles, searching for hidden resources, or finding creative ways to adapt when things don't go as planned.

I hope your healthcare journey is smooth sailing, but even if you have access to the best care possible, there's a chance you'll still run into tough times along the way. It's during those moments that you'll need to channel your inner "comeback kid" and tap into your "can-do" spirit, even when it feels like you're running on fumes.

Let me share a quick story that captures what I've learned about facing challenges, accepting help, and remembering that being seen and supported on our own terms is the essence of good care and of being human.

I once joined a group of friends for ice skating. I showed up with so much confidence, even though I needed a cane to walk. After renting the skates, I put them on and tried to stand, only to almost fall over. But I didn't. I hobbled over to the rink with my cane in one hand, looking out for anything I could find to hold on to. Once I got to the rink, I grabbed the rail and tapped the blade of my skate on the ice to see how slippery it was. Turns out, it was very slippery. The only thing that would have made it more slippery is a banana peel. I felt defeated before I'd even started.

I turned to leave the rink when I heard a friend call out my name. She asked where I was going, and I explained that while I'd thought that I might be able to make it out on the ice, it wasn't going to work out. She reached out her hands and said, "Grab on to me if you want, and we'll skate together."

It turns out, she was once a competitive figure skater. She skated backwards while pulling me around the rink. I was terrified, but I also laughed the whole time.

There are three lessons from that day. First of all, ice skating is not my strong suit. Second, when you want something badly enough, you have to try. Do what's within your control, even if it feels impossible. The best way to know how your story will end is to be the one writing it. Finally, difficult circumstances and joy can exist at the same time. Even when life is hard, you can choose joy.

I'd be lying if I said I've never wondered, "Why me?" Early on, it just felt so unfair. But then I saw an interview with baseball great Darryl Strawberry, who'd been diagnosed with cancer. When asked if he ever thought, "Why me?" he replied, "Why *not* me?" That hit me hard. His response reminded me that no one is immune to tough times. We're all human. That perspective helped me focus on what I could do, not just what I'd lost. I couldn't change what had happened, but I could control how I responded. Strawberry's message of acceptance boosted my drive and helped me keep moving forward.

Experiencing a health crisis or living with a disability doesn't mean you can't have an incredible life. Yes, there will be unique challenges, but there will also be opportunities for growth, resilience, and discovering your true strength. In the end, it's not about the obstacles we face but how we face them and who we invite to skate alongside us. That's what allows us to live our best lives, and that's the heart of person-centered care.

NINE

SHOW ME THE MONEY

(AND THROW IN SOME PERKS)

Navigating the U.S. healthcare system is pretty straightforward—said no one ever.

Before I dive in, I want to manage expectations. This chapter is not offered as a deep policy or financial analysis. It's a patient's exploration fueled by the curiosity and frustrations of someone trying to make sense of the healthcare system.

When I think about person-centered care, I think about problem-solving with my doctor, or even implementing strategies to make my home safer. But my healthcare experience is also shaped by a backstory of policies, financial pressures, and insurance structures.

Some of these administrative elements help ease burdens and make access to care smoother, while others can create significant hurdles. These challenges are more than just inconveniences—they can have a direct impact on whether care is prompt, respectful, and truly person-centered.

While I'm still learning the details, I know that these complexities can create barriers to accessing care that honors each person's needs, values, and preferences. The health insurance landscape in the United States is constantly evolving, and new policies can make an already complex system even harder to navigate. This ongoing uncertainty affects everyone, from those seeking routine care to people facing significant health challenges. This instability and confusion can make it difficult to access services that support a person-centered approach.

Many people who rely on marketplace coverage, and some who rely on Medicare or Medicaid, can be especially vulnerable to policy changes when navigating the system without the structured support that managed care often provides. For anyone, managing health insurance alone can make person-centered care feel harder to reach. Staying informed about these changes and sharing concerns with policymakers isn't just about managing benefits. It helps champion a fundamental component that makes person-centered care possible.

Now, I'll admit: this chapter isn't flashy. There are no dramatic reveals—don't expect me to start tap dancing. But I've learned that looking behind the curtain at how money flows and what shapes care delivery has completely changed how I think about healthcare. The information I share here is based on sources I reviewed as of 2025. I've aimed to be thorough, but some relevant studies may not be included.

Also, keep in mind that details, like healthcare costs, coverage rules, and statistics, can vary widely depending on where you live, your insurer, when the data were collected, and even the data source. That's why it's important to check with your insurer (and, when relevant, your provider or local resources) for the most current, accurate, and relevant information for your situation.

I used to complain about the high cost of healthcare and annoying complications (okay, I still do), but now I also have a *slightly* better understanding of the underlying structure that fuels those frustrations. This chapter isn't meant to provide a detailed financial breakdown, but to highlight key patterns and insights I've encountered as a patient navigating today's healthcare system.

Whether you work in the industry or are simply trying to understand how it all fits together, consider this a window into one patient's journey to decipher how the system really works. There's much more to learn than what I've covered here, so I hope you'll stay curious, keep digging, share your insights with others, and always advocate for the care you deserve.

THE COST OF HEALTHCARE IN THE UNITED STATES

The United States spends a significant amount of money on healthcare. According to the Centers for Medicare and Medicaid Services (as reported by the Kaiser Family Foundation), total national healthcare expenditures rose from an estimated $1.4 trillion in 2000 to $4.9 trillion in 2023, a 250% increase.[1] In 2023, the U.S. spent about 17% of its GDP on healthcare, while other high-income countries typically spent between 8% and 12%, based on Organisation for Economic Co-operation and Development data cited by the Commonwealth Fund.[2]

Despite these substantial investments and access to advanced medical expertise and technology, U.S. health outcomes consistently rank last or near the bottom among comparable nations.[3] However, I believe that by embracing a more person-centered approach to healthcare—one that inherently fosters safety, considers social drivers, and prioritizes overall well-being— patients, providers, and payers together can help shift this trajectory.

To build a healthcare system that truly works for people, positive health outcomes—not just money—must be at the center of how we measure value.

THE BUSINESS OF HEALTHCARE: MARGINS, OVERHEAD, AND PATIENT CARE

I always assumed that the health insurance industry had a high profit margin. In reality, data show that U.S. health insurers' net profit margins in recent years have generally ranged from below 1% to around 3%.[4] As with any business, health insurance companies also have administrative expenses. These costs cover functions like claims processing, customer service, member outreach and engagement, and other operations associated with running the business. Industry data put these expenses at approximately 16.4%.[5] Traditional Medicare spends about 1.3% on administrative costs.[6] In general, streamlined administration, standardized benefits, and a lack of marketing and profit-driven expenses can help contain costs.

And it's not just health insurance companies that have administration costs. Healthcare settings also have administrative expenses. One analysis found that for-profit hospitals spend about 20.5% of their expenses on administration, nonprofit hospitals not affiliated with a religion spend approximately 17.7%, and government hospitals spend roughly 16.2%, though individual hospitals can vary widely.[7] Despite these differences, a systematic review examining quality of care by ownership type found no consistent evidence that for-profit hospitals provide better quality care than other types.[8]

Regardless of ownership, one thing is clear: paperwork extends beyond the front desk. Doctors often carry that burden, too. Some administrative tasks in healthcare settings, like negotiating with insurance companies, completing prior authorizations, and managing billing paperwork, are essential to delivering person-centered care but don't always require the extensive medical training physicians undergo. Yet many doctors carry the burden of these responsibilities, leaving less time to spend with patients. Call me overly attached, possessive, or just plain jealous, but I want doctors to be in a relationship with their patients, not their paperwork.

It can also be difficult for patients to deal with insurance companies. Still, there are people inside those organizations who genuinely want to help members and try to cut through the red tape to speed up access to care and reduce administrative inefficiencies (remember how Mr. Rogers told kids to look for the helpers?). They may not control how the system was built, but they often know how it works. Recognizing and leaning on those helpers can make a real difference.

At the same time, zooming out beyond individual experience reveals a broader picture: how healthcare dollars are spent, and the policies and priorities that shape patient care. In the U.S., we navigate a multi-payer system made up of private insurance, employer plans, and public programs like Medicare and Medicaid—all delivered through a mix of for-profit and non-profit providers. These structures influence how care is delivered and what drives decisions. Examining the business behind healthcare hasn't just enhanced my knowledge; it's made me more confident as I speak up for person-centered care.

PILLS, PRICES, AND PATIENT PAINS

One of the biggest barriers to healthcare for many Americans is the high cost of prescription drugs. A RAND analysis found that, on average, U.S. prices were 2.78 times higher than those in other countries, with brand-name drugs costing more than four times as much.[9] Credible media outlets are amplifying significant price gaps in common life-saving drugs. For example, Forbes reported that when the hepatitis C treatment, Sovaldi, launched in the U.S., it was priced at about $84,000 for a full course. The generic versions of Sovaldi were available in India for less than $1,000. Similarly, the EpiPen has been reported to cost more than $600 for a two-pack in the U.S. compared to about $70 in the U.K.[10]

Rising drug costs can impact how Americans manage their care. A U.S. poll shows that more than half of Americans worry about affording prescriptions, and about three in ten report skipping doses, cutting pills, or avoiding filling prescriptions due to cost.[11]

While pharmaceutical innovation has produced groundbreaking treatments, launch prices for new drugs in the U.S. continue to escalate. The median annual list price rose from about $2,100 in 2008 to well over $180,000 by 2021, with nearly half of 2020–2021 approvals priced above $150,000 per year.[12] By 2024, that number rose to $370,000.[13] This is especially concerning for patients with rare illnesses or those needing costly specialty biologics, which are often life-saving but unaffordable for many.

It's hard to appreciate new and innovative medicines when their high prices put them out of reach. Real lives are at stake, and the financial strain of prescription drugs not only threatens health outcomes but can also add significant stress to patients and families. We *must* figure out a systemic solution to make prescription drugs and overall healthcare costs more affordable for everyone.

COBRA: BENEFITS, BUMPS, AND BLIPS

After my spinal cord surgery, I relied on COBRA—the U.S. law known as the Consolidated Omnibus Budget Reconciliation Act—to keep my health coverage. At the time, it was relatively affordable. Even without online payments, paying the premium was a straightforward process. These days, though, COBRA feels more like an acronym for *Confusing Outdated Bureaucracy Raising Anxiety* (my unofficial take, don't tell anyone).

Although online bill payment is now standard, some COBRA administrators haven't kept up. During a more recent experience, I paid my health insurance premium online and had a smooth experience. But I was required to mail a check for dental and vision coverage. In 2025, there was no online portal to check my balance for this particular provider, and none of my mailed statements reflected recent payments, making it hard to track what I owed.

Outdated processes add unnecessary stress and confusion when clear, accessible information is most needed. They can also lead to missed payments and coverage lapses, putting health at serious risk. I hadn't fully realized how much administrative systems impact both the cost and quality of care. For the U.S. healthcare system to truly serve patients, these processes must evolve and improve.

HIDDEN GEMS: OPPORTUNITIES WITHIN THE SYSTEM

Part of effective problem-solving is recognizing my own gaps in perspective. While I've given a lot of headspace to my frustrations about the healthcare system, I've also discovered unexpected opportunities and resources that can support my health journey and actively promote a more person-centered approach. Here are a few "hidden gems" often found in health insurance policies that I haven't fully appreciated or have taken for granted:

- **Wellness Programs:** Some insurance policies include programs to help manage stress, improve mental health, boost fitness, quit smoking, and encourage better eating habits. These benefits are designed to proactively support overall well-being.
- **Telehealth and 24/7 Medical Advice:** More health insurance plans are offering easy access to telehealth consultations—sometimes even round-the-clock nurse hotlines. This can be a convenient option for quick questions or after-hours concerns.
- **Patient Advocacy Services:** Some insurers and employers provide dedicated patient advocates to help navigate claims, appeals, and tricky coverage questions. Since very few people appeal coverage denials, this kind of support could play a key role in resolving issues effectively.
- **Feedback Opportunities:** Many healthcare facilities and insurance companies administer surveys to gather information to inform patient experience. Even if they don't offer a $5.00 gift card for a cup of coffee to participate, your input just might lead to better patient experiences for all of us.
- **Annual Wellness Visits:** Included in many policies, these visits are essential for preventive care and catching health concerns early. Remembering to schedule and attend these checkups is one of the most impactful actions for long-term health.

- **Online Tools and Apps:** Web portals and mobile apps can help you track claims, benefits, and healthcare spending in real time, streamlining the administrative side of healthcare.
- **Second Opinions:** Some insurance plans cover or even encourage second opinions for complex diagnoses or major procedures. Many aspects of medicine involve both art and science, so it's worth checking your coverage if you think another perspective could help.
- **Discounts on Alternative Therapies:** Many policies now offer discounts or partial coverage for services like acupuncture or chiropractic care—just pay attention to network requirements to ensure coverage applies.

For many, these hidden gems are within reach and can make a real difference if activated. They're like finding money in your jacket pocket—a welcome surprise that can make your day.

PROMISES WORTH WATCHING

In June 2025, AHIP, the national trade association representing health insurance companies in the U.S., announced a series of new voluntary commitments from insurers aimed at improving the experience of both patients and healthcare providers.[14] The goal is to provide faster, more direct access to necessary treatments and services while easing administrative burdens, such as those mentioned earlier in this chapter, that often complicate care.

New commitments by the health insurance industry are also intended to support providers by streamlining prior authorization processes, making them more efficient, transparent, and aligned with evidence-based care. Some of these actions include standardizing electronic prior authorization, ensuring continuity of care when patients switch insurance plans, and improving communication and transparency around coverage decisions.

These commitments are a step in the right direction and an important acknowledgment from the insurance industry that it can do better. If implemented fully, these commitments have the potential to better position patients to experience more person-centered care. They also create an accountability mechanism by giving us something to expect, and something to push for, whether we're dealing with insurance companies or reaching out to the policy-makers who help shape how those companies operate. If we want a healthcare system that's more responsive, more coordinated, and truly centered on people, then follow-through on these promises is key.

MOVING FORWARD

WITH PERSON-CENTERED CARE

Person-centered care goes beyond personal commitment or even the best of intentions. If you've ever made a New Year's resolution, you know what I mean—it's easy to commit, but much harder to follow through without anticipating obstacles or having a clear sense of direction. Throughout this book, I've highlighted a host of barriers that can hinder the delivery of person-centered care, such as financial constraints, administrative hurdles, and poor communication.

As a highly regulated industry, health insurance operates under rigid policies, some of which are designed to protect patients and ensure compliance with regulatory requirements. At the same time, the combination of strict policies, time constraints, fragmented systems, limited training, and scarce organizational resources can make it difficult for even the most dedicated patients, providers, and payers to apply person-centered principles in practice.

As I close this book, my goal is to inspire action. One conceptual framework on person-centered care underscores the importance of professional training and education to equip staff with the skills to elicit patient narratives, build genuine partnerships, and document shared goals. Just as essential are strong leadership, organizational support, and engaging patients as active partners in their care, including co-creating care plans—approaches shown to improve both implementation and outcomes.[1] Together, these strategies can help bridge the gap between the ideal and the reality of person-centered care.

Putting Care into Action For A Person-Centered Future

Over the years, I've learned that navigating a serious health condition and thriving while living with a disability require more than medical breakthroughs or personal grit. It takes a system where everyone plays a role: patients, providers, and payers, each with their own responsibilities and opportunities to make care more person-centered.

Drawing on my personal experiences, frameworks that guide person-centered care, and the shared wisdom of others with personal and professional experience in healthcare, I've gathered the practical strategies I wish I'd known from the very beginning. Some insights reach back to my initial AVM diagnosis, while others reflect recent advancements that were unimaginable at the start of my journey.

I share these insights in the spirit of serving as a thought partner to spark ideas and offer encouragement as you work to advance person-centered care. I recognize that not everything will apply to every reader or setting. Some items may already be part of your daily practice, some may serve as friendly reminders, some may just be informative, and others might be new ideas waiting to be explored.

You'll find abbreviated lists just below. For those seeking more detail, I have included expanded versions with brief introductions in the appendices at the end of the book.

Abbreviated List of Insights for Patients (See Appendix B for the expanded list)

- **Listen to Your Body:** Pain and other symptoms may signal important health issues. Work with your doctor to understand the underlying cause. Review treatment options together and discuss potential side effects. This approach focuses on relieving discomfort while also identifying and addressing the underlying cause, rather than just masking symptoms.
- **Document Interactions:** Record names, dates, and key points from conversations with providers, insurers, and others involved in your care. Note anyone who was especially helpful for future assistance or when giving feedback to reinforce your vision of quality care.
- **Engage in Shared Decision-Making**: When undergoing care, discuss all options, risks, and benefits with your doctor. Share the reasons behind your preferences and ask your doctor to explain the rationale for any recommendations. Let your doctor know about any changes you'd like to try, so you can work together to ensure your safety.
- **Get to Know Your Coverage:** Review your health insurance policy to understand your benefits, how to access urgent care and specialists in your network, your financial responsibilities, and the appeals process. As a practice exercise, make a list of questions and contact your insurer for answers. This will help you become

more familiar with your coverage and can make it easier to access information and care when you need it.

- **Check Your Medical Records for Accuracy**: Review your doctor's notes, medication lists, and test results to ensure they are specific and accurately reflect your care and concerns. Notify your provider if any information is missing, vague, or incorrect.

- **Consider Naming an Authorized Representative:** If you need help navigating health insurance or managing hospital-related tasks, consider naming a trusted family member, friend, caregiver, or legal representative as an "authorized representative" to handle certain matters on your behalf. You may need to submit an authorization form.

- **Learn to Distinguish Between Helpful and Harmful Information**: Promote your safety by asking providers for strategies to identify trustworthy resources, recognize warning signs of unreliable information, and know when to be suspicious about health advice.

- **Stay Informed on AI-Enhanced Screening:** Ask your provider about innovative tools like AI-assisted screenings that analyze medical data to detect health risks, sometimes even before symptoms appear. Discuss how accurate they are for someone with your personal health profile and weigh the potential benefits and limitations.

- **Support Caregivers**: Be mindful of signs of caregiver burnout, such as exhaustion, stress, or feeling overwhelmed, and consider respite services or support resources to help maintain your caregiver's well-being.

- **Address Emotional Needs**: Explore counseling or support groups to help manage your mental health and enhance your overall well-being as needed.

Abbreviated List of Insights for Providers (See Appendix C for the expanded list)

- **Establish Clear Protocols Around Patient Engagement:** Ensure all team members are equipped and empowered to identify and address safety, quality, and ethical concerns that impact the patient experience and outcomes.
- **Promote Safety Awareness**: Inform patients about safety features such as emergency call buttons, handrails, non-slip flooring, and fall-prevention protocols that help create a secure environment. Share how the facility upholds clinical safety by managing medications, preventing infections, and ensuring accurate patient identification and appropriate care.
- **Provide Patient Education Resources**: Ensure access to evidence-based education materials and support for self-care at every stage of care, including after discharge. Help patients understand how to evaluate resources to identify credible sources and recognize those that may be questionable or harmful.
- **Foster Transparency:** Use plain language to explain conditions, treatments, processes, and potential side effects or risks. Seek to understand patients' concerns and uncertainties and offer alternative approaches when appropriate.

- **Practice Shared Decision-Making:** Explain the importance of evidence-based options and consider alternative approaches suggested by patients. For all treatment options, discuss possible risks and side effects in plain language, and collaborate with the patient to select the best fit.
- **Reflect and Evolve:** Develop and use strategies to regularly reflect on your interactions with patients to foster self-awareness and more productive patient engagement. Encourage your colleagues to do the same.
- **Empower and Support Caregivers:** Provide caregivers with written guidance and ongoing support to help them effectively manage the patient's care and prevent burnout. Use regular check-ins and teach-back methods to confirm their understanding and reinforce a collaborative partnership.
- **Promote Provider Well-Being:** Address burnout, foster resilience, and cultivate a culture that supports empathy and maintains high-quality, safe care among providers by supporting strategies such as peer support, mindfulness, workload management, and safe working conditions.
- **Stay Current with Technology**: Help patients identify and select technologies that support their care, independence, and overall well-being. These may include assistive devices, AI-powered solutions, and commonly available tools like smartphone apps and built-in device features.
- **Monitor Billing Accuracy:** Reduce delays in care and the loss of provider time and revenue caused by billing errors. Regularly assess procedures, ensure claims are

accurate and complete, and provide ongoing training to minimize denials.

Abbreviated List of Insights for Payers (See Appendix D for the expanded list)

- **Streamline Approval Processes:** Simplify and accelerate review procedures to avoid unnecessary delays for urgent or specialist care. Clearly communicate steps, timelines, and decision criteria to patients and providers in plain language and through digital channels. When possible, use care navigators or support staff to promote transparency and build trust in the process.
- **Support Individualized Claims Assessments:** Prioritize prompt reviews of medically justified requests, especially for out-of-network care or exceptions. Ensure decisions are guided by the treating provider's clinical judgment, rather than solely by administrative criteria, to uphold safe, personalized care.
- **Prioritize Clear Communication:** Share specific, evidence-based criteria and real-world examples used in authorization decisions. Provide clear, plain-language explanations for approvals or denials, along with step-by-step guidance on how to appeal or resubmit when needed.
- **Provide Caregiver Support**: Offer resources, helplines, and educational materials to empower caregivers. Consider covering caregiver training and respite services to support caregiver well-being, promote continuity of care, and improve outcomes for both caregivers and those they support.

- **Promote Interoperability**: Champion universal compatibility between medical records, claims databases, and document systems so all providers and patients can easily share and access essential health information, regardless of software vendor.
- **Share Denial Trends with Providers:** Develop systems that analyze and share denial trends to help providers understand why claims are being denied. Include mechanisms to disaggregate data by provider and offer this information as needed to support process improvement, reduce administrative burden, and improve access to prompt care.
- **Collaborate with Providers on Claims Burden:** Engage directly with clinicians to identify pain points in claims and prior authorization processes. Work together to reduce duplicative paperwork and time spent on medical necessity documentation, enabling providers to focus more on patient care and less on administrative tasks.
- **Expand Feedback Gathering:** In addition to traditional member surveys, seek input from families, providers, colleagues, and community stakeholders. Use informal feedback channels and advisory boards to better understand the needs of people affected by disability and adverse social drivers of health. Include frequent microsurveys to gather quick, real-time feedback and spot emerging issues.
- **Analyze Member Feedback and Implement Change:** Disaggregate member data to identify patterns and gaps in care. Use these insights to inform policy changes and

guide targeted improvements that enhance access, quality, and outcomes for all members.

- **Keep Your Word:** Whether you make a public commitment or a promise to an individual member, always follow through. If unforeseen circumstances such as new regulatory restrictions prevent you from doing so, be transparent about the change and clearly explain why.

LOVE LETTERS

TO PATIENTS, PROVIDERS, AND PAYERS

Can I just say how happy I am that you've made it to the end? I know getting through a book on healthcare can sometimes require more patience than opening a childproof prescription bottle, so I truly appreciate you sticking with me. And hey, if you happened to pop in and out, no judgment here. I won't tell anyone.

We live in a time when medical breakthroughs are happening faster than ever, but the real challenge is ensuring healthcare delivery actually helps people benefit from those advances. Too often, good healthcare is technically available, but still out of reach. That's why I'm such a fan of a person-centered approach. A healthcare system that supports person-centered care helps make high-quality, accessible, and affordable service available for everyone it serves.

As I wrap up, I want to leave you with a few "love letters"—one for patients, one for providers, and one for payers. Find the one that fits you best, but feel free to peek at the others (after all, we've made it to the end of the book together, we're practically family now).

Dear Patient,

Whether you're facing routine care or a serious health crisis, you deserve the very best care possible. I know it can be hard to speak up for yourself sometimes—maybe you don't want to be a burden, or you're worried about hearing bad news. Trust me, I've been there too. But remember, the more involved you are in your care, the better your chances of receiving solutions that truly work for you. So ask questions. Give input. Let your preferences be known. And remember, if something doesn't seem right, don't hesitate to speak up—your health and safety are the top priorities.

You don't have to go through your health journey alone. Consider turning to family, trusted friends, or even a patient advocate for support. You'll probably find that there are more people in your corner than you realize—some of them might even bring snacks. And don't forget to show appreciation for the superstars who are holding your hand along the way. That might be someone from your personal support network who's helping you get through this, or even a member of your care team who sees you for the important, unique, and wonderful person you are.

And always remember, I'm by your side—whether I'm on your nightstand, tucked in your backpack, or just hanging out on your bookshelf, leading all your other books in a group cheer just for you. You've got this!

With admiration,
Cynthia

Dear Provider,

First of all, thank you for choosing a profession that helps people. I know we've had our ups and downs, with difficult conversations and lots of negotiations. And sometimes you drop big words that sound like conversational Latin. But at the end of the day, I know we want the same thing—excellent health outcomes (and a little nap from time to time).

The healthcare field is prestigious, but scrubs and medical gloves aside, I know you're operating inside of an industry that doesn't always make things easy. Long hours, endless administrative tasks, and large caseloads must be daunting. By the way, have you eaten?

As a patient, I appreciate the sacrifices you make. It may not always feel obvious, but treating your patients as individuals with unique goals and needs truly makes a difference. Providers who speak with their patients, not at them; who approach the provider-patient relationship as a partnership instead of a dictatorship; and who show genuine empathy—drop the mic—you're making the world easier for a lot of people and building a legacy that would make your grandma proud. And trust me—the impact you have on your patients' lives is significant. You'll be like Taylor Swift with her Swifties—fans will celebrate you for years to come.

So when the admin work piles up and your scissors start to dull from cutting through so much red tape, take a breath, and a bathroom break, and remember how much you matter to the people who need your expertise, care, and compassion. You've got a fan club of patients, both past and present, cheering you on—no autographs required (but a selfie would be nice).

With gratitude,
Cynthia

Dear Payer,

This is a tough letter to write. Is it just me, or is there a wedge in our relationship?

I know we're supposed to be on the same team, but there are times when it feels like you just don't get me. And I'll admit—I don't always understand you either, especially when you send cryptic letters full of codes, but no decoder ring to help me figure things out.

I want to understand you better, but it's hard to get through when I call. Sure, the hold music is relaxing, but I'd rather listen to answers to my questions than Beethoven's Moonlight Sonata. I don't want to seem clingy, but it feels like you're trying to avoid me. Did I do something wrong?

Just like our relationship, the system we operate in is complicated. I'm sure you're juggling challenges I don't always see, and you may not realize how much your decisions affect me. But I'm not giving up on us. I'd love for us to actually talk—like, really talk (maybe even with a counselor, if my plan covers it). I want us to figure out how to work together as a team so I can better understand my plan, maximize my benefits, and manage my health.

Let's put the billing codes and assumptions aside, and put our heads together to focus on what really matters: people's lives. I'll drop the grudges if we collaborate on coverage.

So, Payer... will you accept this rose?

With bated breath,
Cynthia

Here's to all of us shaping the future of healthcare through person-centered care. I'm excited to see what you do next, and I hope you'll keep the *Clear Cane Chronicles* as your sidekick along the way.

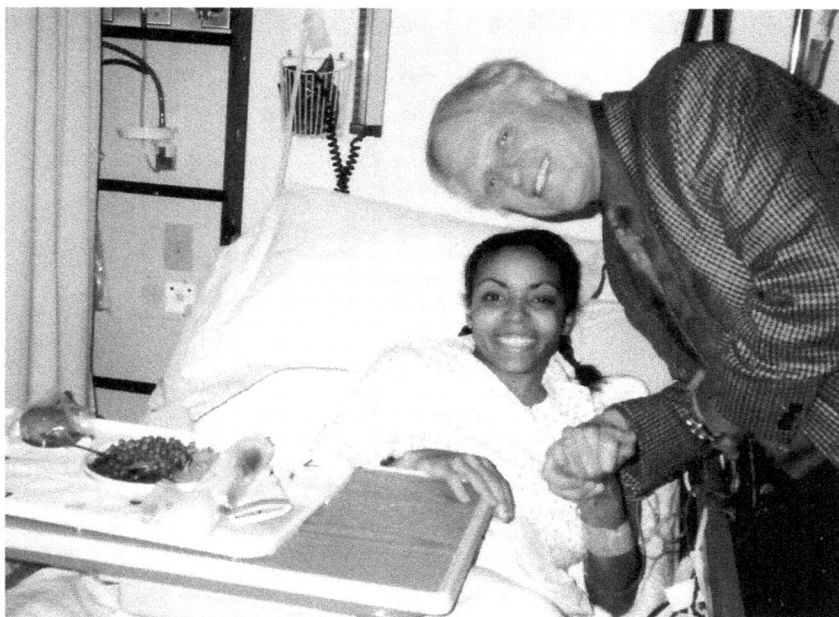

Cynthia and Fred, November 1997

APPENDIX A

FRAMEWORKS ADVANCING
PERSON-CENTERED CARE

Both the Picker Principles of Person Centred Care and the NAB's Six Principles to Modernize the Healthcare Infrastructure frameworks were developed to help transform the concept of exceptional healthcare into reality. They serve as practical tools for patients advocating for better care, support providers in delivering care that truly meets individual needs, and encourage payers to invest in models that put people first. By reflecting on these principles, patients, providers, and payers can play their part in building a healthcare system where every person is seen, heard, and valued as a partner in their own care.

Picker Principles of Person Centred Care

The Picker Institute developed the Picker Principles of Person Centred Care through extensive research and direct engagement with patients, families, and healthcare providers in an effort to understand and share what truly matters to people during their healthcare experiences. Over time, the Picker Institute's framework has evolved from a focus on patient-centered care—centered on the clinical experience—to a broader vision of person-centered care that recognizes the whole person, including their goals, values, relationships, and environment. The principles are used to help guide care that involves patients taking an active role, respecting individual preferences, needs, and values.

The Picker Principles include:

1. **Fast access to reliable healthcare advice.** Access to the right services at the right time is essential for high-quality care that meets individuals' needs. Access includes: ease of scheduling appointments; minimal waiting for referrals or treatment; and availability of appropriate professionals and advice. Fast, easy access is important, both for routine care and unplanned crises.

2. **Effective treatment by trusted professionals.** Positive therapeutic relationships are at the heart of person centred care. People should receive clinically appropriate and effective care that meets their needs and is respectful of their preferences. Interactions with care professionals should inspire a sense of confidence and trust.

3. **Continuity of care and smooth transitions.** Care journeys bring people into contact with a range of providers and staff. Ensuring these transitions are seamless is vital to person-centered, coordinated care. All people should experience continuity in information,

in the relationships they have with staff, and in the way their care is managed.

4. **Involvement and support for family and carers.** Providers and staff must acknowledge the importance of people's families, carers, friends, and wider support networks in their overall health and well-being. Their involvement should be welcomed and supported. The emotional impact of caring responsibilities should not be underestimated: carers need to feel supported throughout.

5. **Clear information, communication, and support for self-care.** People using health and care services should receive reliable, high-quality, and accessible information at every stage in their journey. Information should be provided at appropriate times, in an understandable way, and should support people to make informed decisions and manage their own care.

6. **Involvement in decisions and respect for preferences.** People have the right to be involved in and to make decisions about their health and care. Providers should work with people in equal, reciprocal partnerships, and should respect people's choices and preferences, including but not limited to those that reflect their background, social, and cultural values.

7. **Emotional support, empathy, and respect.** Person-centered care demands a caring and holistic approach. People providing care should show empathy and respect, recognising an individual's emotional needs. For care to be compassionate, it must be delivered with respect, sensitivity, and appreciation of the person as an individual.

8. **Attention to physical and environmental needs.**
   People deserve to be treated and cared for in safe,
   comfortable environments that afford them privacy and
   dignity. Similarly, care professionals should be mindful
   of people's physical needs, including pain management,
   assistance with activities, and personal care.

The Six Principles to Modernize the Healthcare Infrastructure

The National Advisory Board (NAB) on Improving Health-care Services for Older Adults and People with Disabilities developed the Six Principles to Modernize the Healthcare Infrastructure through a consensus-driven process informed by both professional expertise and lived experience. The principles were shaped by a culturally diverse group of advocates, policy leaders, healthcare professionals, and academics, many of whom are individuals with disabilities, older adults, caregivers, or close family members of those navigating long-term care systems. The principles reflect the collective wisdom of people who have spent decades confronting the challenges of a fragmented healthcare system and working to improve access, opportunity, independence, and inclusion for all.

These guiding principles inform policy recommendations aimed at improving long-term services and supports. Beyond shaping policy, the principles serve as a guide for developing and implementing practical strategies that support independence and ensure that older adults and people with disabilities can access excellent, person-centered healthcare tailored to their goals, needs, and circumstances.

Since the original release in 2009, the NAB's six principles were overhauled in 2020 during the 30th anniversary of the ADA to reflect evolving priorities and challenges. As a member of the NAB for roughly ten years, I had the opportunity to contribute to the second version, which is reflected throughout this book.

The Six Principles to Modernize the Healthcare Infrastructure

1. **Improve Health and Well-Being Through Individual Empowerment and System Coordination**. Empower people to manage their health and wellness with their chosen support network, healthcare and service providers, and communities, regardless of a person's condition or perceived capabilities.
2. **Achieve Community Inclusion and Full Participation**. Expedite access, choice, and full integration into meaningful activities of community living (social, economic, educational, and recreational) by providing and coordinating necessary services and supports.
3. **Ensure Full Access to Services and Supports**. Revise and strengthen policies and programs to provide affordable, flexible access to the services and supports people need to live independently.
4. **Value Dignity and Choice**. Valuing and ensuring dignity, personal strengths, and self-determination must be core to successful and sustainable long-term services and supports.
5. **Achieve Access to Meaningful Work and Activities**. Achieve full community participation in valued roles and equitable access to competitive, integrated employment or other meaningful activities.

6. **Accelerate Access to Innovative Technologies**. Ensure that people with disabilities and older adults are key stakeholders and fully involved in the development of new technologies, and have the necessary technologies that support independence, social participation, dignity, and self-direction.

APPENDIX B

EXPANDED LIST OF INSIGHTS FOR PATIENTS

These insights come from lessons learned throughout my healthcare journey. I share them with appreciation for every individual's unique experience, and offer them in the spirit of encouraging reflection.

Consider how to adapt these as needed to fit your circumstances and revisit them as your needs and experiences evolve over time. My hope is that some of these will resonate with you and add value to your life. If any speak to you, I invite you to share them with other patients.

Finally, please remember: I'm sharing what worked for me, based on my lived experience. I'm not a medical professional, and this is not medical advice. Always consult a licensed healthcare provider for guidance tailored to your unique situation. And if at any point you feel unsure or uncomfortable with your current provider, consider seeking a second opinion or speaking with another qualified clinician (and if you love your current provider, tell a friend!).

Self-Advocacy and Empowerment

- **Listen to Your Body:** Pain and other symptoms may signal important health issues. Work with your doctor to understand the underlying cause. Review treatment options together and discuss potential side effects. This approach focuses on relieving discomfort while also identifying and addressing the underlying cause, rather than just masking symptoms.
- **Document Interactions:** Record names, dates, and key points from conversations with providers, insurers, and others involved in your care. Note anyone who was especially helpful for future assistance or when giving feedback to reinforce your vision of quality care.
- **Understand Your Rights**: Ask your healthcare provider or facility for information about your patient rights, including how your personal information is protected, what to expect during your care, and how to participate in treatment decisions. Inquire about the proper channels for expressing concerns, such as patient advocates, ombuds offices, or regulatory agencies.
- **Foster Clear Communication:** Speak up about your concerns, ask questions, and request explanations in plain language and formats that you understand and without jargon. For added clarity and to keep a record, consider following up important conversations in writing.
- **Learn to Distinguish Between Helpful and Harmful Information**: Promote your safety by asking providers for strategies to identify trustworthy resources, recognize

warning signs of unreliable information, and know when to be suspicious about health advice.

- **Report Concerns:** Notify providers or advocates about safety issues, access needs, unfair treatment, or inappropriate behavior.
- **Assert Your Rights**: Seek resources such as those offered through The Joint Commission's "Know Your Rights" campaign to develop strategies to voice concerns.
- **Use Trusted Resources**: Ask your provider for evidence-based patient information and well-vetted, credible AI-powered tools to help you understand your condition and treatment options.
- **Be Resourceful**: Stay proactive in pursuing the best care for your health. Explore all available options—get a second opinion, file an insurance appeal, ask about clinical trials, or look into other avenues that meet your needs.
- **Engage with Elected Officials**: Urge your representatives to prioritize accessible, affordable, and quality healthcare. Share your personal experiences and support policies that promote positive health outcomes for everyone.

Insurance and Financial Considerations

- **Get to Know Your Coverage:** Review your health insurance policy to understand your benefits, how to access urgent care and specialists in your network, your financial responsibilities, and the appeals process. As a practice exercise, make a list of questions and contact

CYNTHIA OVERTON, PHD

your insurer for answers. This will help you become more familiar with your coverage and can make it easier to access information and care when you need it.

- **Understand Non-Approvals:** Learn the difference between claim denials, holds, requests for information, and other terms used when coverage isn't approved, so you're better prepared to take the next step and avoid unnecessary delays.
- **Ask About Costs**: Before receiving medical care, inquire about expected costs, available payment options, and financial assistance programs. Consider cost-saving strategies like negotiating fees, requesting lower interest rates, and arranging a payment plan.
- **Look Into Support Programs:** If a medical condition impacts your ability to work, explore eligibility requirements for job-protected leave under the Family and Medical Leave Act (FMLA), as well as for Social Security disability benefits, state rehabilitation services, community resources, and other support programs. Approach paperwork with persistence and care, and don't hesitate to reach out for assistance if you need help.

Managing Your Care

- **Plan for Unexpected Changes**: Prepare ahead by making sure you and your emergency contacts understand what steps to take if you get ill or your condition worsens, and keep contact information for everyone involved in your care easily accessible. Have a clear backup plan in place so you're ready to respond quickly if things don't go as expected.

- **Access Digital Tools**: Explore how patient portals, telemedicine options, and hotlines can help you track your health information and quickly access support and guidance. If you're unsure how to use these tools, look for online tutorials or ask others for help from a trusted family member, friend, or support representative from your provider or insurance company.
- **Manage Your Recovery**: Build skills such as wound care, therapeutic exercises, or using medical equipment to support your recovery and independence. Be sure to receive proper training on how to use equipment safely, and ensure you have access to the devices and supplies required for your care.
- **Monitor and Report Secondary Conditions**: Monitor and promptly tell your provider about any risks related to your condition, such as wounds, infections, or falls.
- **Report Changes in Daily Living**: Let your provider know about any changes to your caregiver or Direct Care Worker (DCW) support, or updates to your living arrangements, so they can adjust your care plan as needed.
- **Stay Current with Preventive Care**: Keep a schedule of recommended screenings, wellness visits, and immunizations as appropriate.
- **Avoid Information Gaps:** During team transitions, ask thorough questions to ensure nothing is overlooked or assumed.

Enlisting Support from Others

- **Seek Support**: Ask for help from family, friends, or members of your faith or community networks. When managing complicated health conditions, consider designating someone who can coordinate your support team and designate tasks such as driving you to appointments and providing meals. Consider enlisting advocacy or ombuds services when navigating business issues becomes overwhelming. Counseling or peer support may be able to help with emotional issues.

- **Support Caregivers**: Be mindful of signs of caregiver burnout, such as exhaustion, stress, or feeling overwhelmed, and consider respite services or support resources to help maintain your caregiver's well-being.

- **Consider Naming an Authorized Representative:** If you need help navigating health insurance or managing hospital-related tasks, consider naming a trusted family member, friend, caregiver, or legal representative as an "authorized representative" to handle certain matters on your behalf. You may need to submit an authorization form.

- **Document Your Intentions:** Write down your care preferences and share them with those involved in your care to ensure your wishes are clear and respected if you're unable to communicate them yourself. Living wills and healthcare proxies help clarify your plans for unexpected situations.

Effective Communication with Providers

- **Engage in Shared Decision-Making**: When undergoing care, discuss all options, risks, and benefits with your doctor. Share the reasons behind your preferences and ask your doctor to explain the rationale for any recommendations. Let your doctor know about any changes you'd like to try, so you can work together to ensure your safety.
- **Ask for Clarity**: Ask questions and request explanations and materials in plain language when engaging with your provider, reviewing documents, or accessing patient information and resources.
- **Monitor and Report Changes:** Use a health journal or tracking app to record symptoms, side effects, and patterns over time. Share updates with your provider promptly, especially if something worsens or feels new.
- **Express Your Needs and Preferences:** Inform your care team about needs related to values, culture, and emotions, such as modesty requirements, dietary restrictions, or access to a quiet space for prayer or reflection. Having this information recorded in your file supports continuity and better care across all your visits.
- **Provide Feedback**: Share your experience by responding to surveys or feedback requests. Your input helps providers and payers understand what's working, what isn't, and directs ongoing improvement for you and others.
- **Communicate with Your Surgeon:** For major surgeries, request a brief pre-op meeting if needed. Prepare your questions and key information in advance.

If a meeting isn't possible or would delay the procedure, and you choose to move forward with this surgeon, share questions and concerns in writing.

- **Explore Adaptation and Rehabilitation Options**: Ask about therapy and adaptive skills training to help you maintain or regain independence and successfully manage new challenges.
- **Stay Informed on AI-Enhanced Screening:** Ask your provider about innovative tools like AI-assisted screenings that analyze medical data to detect health risks, sometimes even before symptoms appear. Discuss how accurate they are for someone with your personal health profile and weigh the potential benefits and limitations.

Care Logistics

- **Organize Your Healthcare Records**: Keep your medical documents organized and easily accessible so you always have the information you need to make informed decisions about your care.
- **Check Your Medical Records for Accuracy**: Review your doctor's notes, medication lists, and test results to ensure they are specific and accurately reflect your care and concerns. Notify your provider if any information is missing, vague, or incorrect.
- **Prepare for Appointments**: Maximize your time with your provider by bringing a list of questions, a way to take notes, and, if helpful, a trusted friend or family member to support you.

- **Activate Your Support Network:** Invite family and friends to join you in social activities and, if you wish, to be involved in your medical care to support your well-being and recovery.
- **Request Disability Accommodations**: Let your provider know before your appointment if you need any accommodations, such as accessible exam rooms, sign language interpreters, or extra time to ensure you can fully access the care you need.
- **Facilitate Smooth Transitions**: When moving between providers or facilities, confirm your follow-up plan, what to do if complications occur, and that your records are transferred appropriately.
- **Manage Medication:** Maintain an up-to-date list of all your medications, including vitamins and supplements. Double-check prescriptions, instructions, and warning labels to ensure safe and correct use. Don't hesitate to follow up with your pharmacist or healthcare professional if you have any questions.
- **Explore Financial and Healthcare Support Options**: If your health condition interferes with your ability to work, check eligibility for local, state, or federal programs for temporary or long-term financial and healthcare support.

Emotional Well-Being, Community, and Inclusion

- **Address Emotional Needs**: Explore counseling or support groups to help manage your mental health and enhance your overall well-being as needed.

- **Engage in Meaningful Activities**: Stay connected and fulfilled by participating in activities that align with your interests and values, and that bring you joy.
- **Socialize**: Stay engaged by connecting with mentors, support groups, organizations, friends, and family.
- **Explore Accommodations**: Request supports through disability services, human resources (HR), or other appropriate channels when returning to work, school, or other settings.
- **Consider Innovative Technology**: Explore how devices powered by artificial intelligence (AI), such as smart wheelchairs, canes, and walkers, virtual assistants, and platforms for social connection or support, can help advance recovery, independence, safety, and social engagement.
- **Protect Your Privacy with Technology:** When using AI-powered devices, apps, or online health platforms, be aware of how your personal health information is collected, stored, and shared. Review privacy settings carefully, and ask your providers or tech support about data security to help safeguard your information.
- **Develop a Wellness Routine**: Work with your care team to discuss and plan nutrition, exercise, and overall wellness strategies.
- **Take Advantage of Community Resources**: Reach out to support and advocacy organizations for assistance and resources.
- **Take Time to Recharge**: Seek out activities that bring you happiness and extend compassion to yourself and those who care for you.

APPENDIX C

As someone without a medical background, I don't know all the clinical details or daily complexities across care settings. My insights are informed by what has helped me as a patient, and are offered with deep respect for all providers, whether you work in a hospital, an independent practice, or any other healthcare setting. I understand that not every item will apply to every provider, depending on specialty, setting, and other factors, but I hope they still resonate and inspire reflection.

Access, Communication & Care Transitions

- **Establish Clear Protocols Around Patient Engagement:** Ensure all team members are equipped and empowered to identify and address safety, quality, and ethical concerns that impact the patient experience and outcomes.

- **Manage Expectations**: When engaging with patients and families, explain wait times, provide interim guidance, and offer reassurance when immediate answers aren't possible.
- **Anticipate Information Bottlenecks:** Collaborate with colleagues and use digital tools such as patient portals, secure messaging, and automated reminders to keep patients informed and engaged about test results, referrals, and other important information.
- **Foster Transparency:** Use plain language to explain conditions, treatments, processes, and potential side effects or risks. Seek to understand patients' concerns and uncertainties and offer alternative approaches when appropriate.
- **Support Shared Understanding:** Whenever possible, document clinical findings with specificity rather than abbreviations like "WNL" to promote accurate communication across care teams, support patient understanding, and help prevent safety issues caused by misinterpretation or delays in diagnosis and treatment.
- **Ensure Continuity and Clarity During Care Transitions:** Before transfers, inform patients of the steps you've taken to support safe, consistent care. Explain the reasons for the transfer, what to expect during the transition, and who will be responsible for each aspect of care. Review key information directly with the patient rather than assuming another provider has done so—this might include risks, side effects, and care details. Follow up with the patient and the next care team to promote a safe, seamless transition.

Person-Centered Relationships & Shared Decision-Making

- **Combine Expertise with Empathy**: Cultivate self-awareness to recognize and address preconceived notions, and use this understanding to provide respectful, high-quality care to every patient.
- **Factor in the Whole Person:** Recognize how patients' values, beliefs, and life circumstances affect their engagement in care. Tailor communication and care plans to align with these factors, fostering trust, collaboration, and improved health outcomes.
- **Build Trust**: Listen attentively to patients, support them through challenging decisions, and consistently follow through on commitments.
- **Practice Shared Decision-Making:** Explain the importance of evidence-based options and consider alternative approaches suggested by patients. For all treatment options, discuss possible risks and side effects in plain language, and collaborate with the patient to select the best fit.
- **Empower Patients**: Encourage patients to ask questions and advocate for themselves. Provide evidence-based, user-friendly information to help them understand their condition and treatment options.
- **Respect Patient Wishes**: After clearly communicating prognosis and treatment options, support patients and families in advance care planning to ensure care aligns with their values and preferences, while upholding standards of safe and effective medical care.
- **Reflect and Evolve:** Develop and use strategies to regularly reflect on your interactions with patients to

foster self-awareness and more productive patient engagement. Encourage your colleagues to do the same.

Family, Support Networks & Self-Management

- **Empower and Support Caregivers:** Provide caregivers with written guidance and ongoing support to help them effectively manage the patient's care and prevent burnout. Use regular check-ins and teach-back methods to confirm their understanding and reinforce a collaborative partnership.
- **Communicate Effectively**: Use plain language and avoid medical jargon. Provide patient information in multiple accessible formats and languages. Adapt your approach for people with different communication needs, including those who are deaf, hard of hearing, blind, or have low vision, by using interpreters, assistive technology, or accessible formats, ensuring everyone can understand and participate in their care.
- **Provide Patient Education Resources**: Ensure access to credible education materials and support for self-care at every stage of care, including after discharge. Help patients understand how to evaluate resources to identify credible sources and recognize those that may be questionable or harmful.
- **Promote Caregiver Well-Being:** Acknowledge the emotional and physical challenges caregivers face. Encourage caregivers to practice self-care, access respite services, and participate in support groups to reduce stress, maintain their health, and sustain compassionate care.

Emotional, Physical & Environmental Support

- **Foster Emotional Security:** Create an environment that encourages open communication by acknowledging patient concerns and connecting them with appropriate emotional support resources.
- **Monitor for Mental Health Needs:** Proactively assess and address depression, anxiety, grief, and other mental health concerns throughout care.
- **Promote Provider Well-Being:** Address burnout, foster resilience, and cultivate a culture that supports empathy and maintains high-quality, safe care among providers by supporting strategies such as peer support, mindfulness, workload management, and safe working conditions.
- **Communicate Accessibility Features**: Inform patients about accessibility features as needed (e.g., ramps, adaptive equipment, Braille, and tactile signage). Let them know how to request accommodations, and remind staff to proactively discuss these options with patients so that everyone can access the care they need.
- **Promote Safety Awareness**: Inform patients about safety features such as emergency call buttons, handrails, non-slip flooring, and fall-prevention protocols that help create a secure environment. Share how the facility upholds clinical safety by managing medications, preventing infections, and ensuring accurate patient identification and appropriate care.

Coordination, Community & Innovation

- **Coordinate Across Services**: Work with medical, social, and community services to ensure comprehensive support both in and out of the clinical setting.
- **Close Health Gaps:** Take proactive steps to identify and eliminate health disparities throughout diagnosis, treatment, and recovery. When using AI and other technologies, ensure data and algorithms represent the diverse populations you serve and actively monitor for unintended bias in their use.
- **Encourage Meaningful Activities**: Learn what is important to each patient and support engagement in activities that reflect their individual interests and values.
- **Stay Current with Technology:** Help patients identify and select technologies that support their care, independence, and overall well-being. These may include assistive devices, AI-powered solutions, and commonly available tools like smartphone apps and built-in device features.

Holistic Care

- **Consider Social Drivers of Health:** Take into account patients' social and environmental factors (e.g., housing stability, access to reliable transportation, food security) when creating care plans to ensure personalized, effective care.
- **Collaborate with Colleagues**: Partner regularly with colleagues from various specialties and locations to

address patients' holistic needs and prevent secondary conditions.

- **Minimize Social Isolation**: Be alert to the ways medical conditions can lead to social isolation and take proactive steps to help prevent this outcome.
- **Respect Individual Needs**: Accommodate dietary restrictions, routines, cultural practices, and religious needs in ways that align with the quality and safety of care.
- **Provide Respectful End-of-Life Care**: Honor patient values and preferences throughout the care journey, including during the transition from active treatment to end-of-life care.

Quality Improvement & System Change

- **Seek Feedback from Patients and Families:** Use plain-language surveys, micro-surveys, and digital tools to gather real-time input. Monitor social media reviews for themes, and engage focus groups or advisory committees with attention to privacy and accessibility.
- **Analyze Feedback and Implement Change:** Track feedback for patterns that reveal strengths and gaps. Use findings to update systems, reduce barriers, and improve care. Follow up when input warrants a direct response.
- **Review and Update Care Plans:** Regularly revisit care plans with patients and families, and update them as needed.
- **Protect Patient Privacy**: Ensure that workflow pressures, physical layout, communication challenges, or

other factors do not compromise privacy and confidentiality requirements.

- **Monitor Billing Accuracy:** Reduce delays in care and the loss of provider time and revenue caused by billing errors. Regularly assess procedures, ensure claims are accurate and complete, and provide ongoing training to minimize denials.

APPENDIX D

EXPANDED LIST OF INSIGHTS FOR PAYERS

Given that insurance companies routinely collect and review member feedback, I understand that many of these insights may already be familiar. Still, I hope to reiterate key issues and provide a reference point to support your work. These reflections are informed by my perspective as a patient, and I offer them in the hope that they will support your continued efforts to guide, communicate with, and ensure optimal healthcare for your members.

Access, Approvals & Navigation

- **Modernize Administrative Systems:** Leverage digital platforms to streamline case management, care navigation, coverage approvals, and payment options to reduce administrative load on providers and members.
- **Collaborate with Providers on Claims Burden:** Engage directly with clinicians to identify pain points in claims and prior authorization processes. Work together

to reduce duplicative paperwork and time spent on medical necessity documentation, enabling providers to focus more on patient care and less on administrative tasks.

- **Streamline Approval Processes:** Simplify and accelerate review procedures to avoid unnecessary delays for urgent or specialist care. Clearly communicate steps, timelines, and decision criteria to patients and providers in plain language and through digital channels. When possible, use care navigators or support staff to promote transparency and build trust in the process.
- **Support Individualized Claims Assessments:** Prioritize prompt reviews of medically justified requests, especially for out-of-network care or exceptions. Ensure decisions are guided by the treating provider's clinical judgment, rather than solely by administrative criteria, to uphold safe, personalized care.
- **Prioritize Clear Communication:** Share specific, evidence-based criteria and real-world examples used in authorization decisions. Provide clear, plain-language explanations for approvals or denials, along with step-by-step guidance on how to appeal or resubmit when needed.
- **Train and Empower Staff**: Equip staff to assist members effectively with courtesy and respect, and ensure they do not deflect or delay support.
- **Reduce Misunderstandings:** Clearly distinguish between claim denials, holds, and requests for information so members understand what action is needed, feel encouraged to pursue coverage, and have greater reason to trust the process.

Continuity, Transitions & Family Support

- **Support Care Transitions for Families:** Assist families in navigating changes between care settings, coordinating follow-up appointments, and arranging for necessary equipment or home care to ensure continuity and reduce confusion.
- **Ensure Prompt Access to Essential Services:** Prevent gaps in care by offering prompt access to rehabilitation, home health, and durable medical equipment, supporting safe and effective recovery for all members.
- **Provide Caregiver Support**: Offer resources, helplines, and educational materials to empower caregivers. Consider covering caregiver training and respite services to support caregiver well-being, promote continuity of care, and improve outcomes for both caregivers and those they support.

Communication, Information & Empowerment

- **Offer Case Managers:** Make case management available to members with complex health needs, as well as those who lack support networks or face challenges navigating the healthcare system. Personalized guidance can improve outcomes, reduce frustration, and expand access to prompt, effective care.
- **Empower Members**: Expand access to online portals that use plain language to help members track claims, review benefits, access documents, and find patient education materials. Support adoption among small practices by addressing cost barriers for these tools.

- **Promote Health Literacy:** Help members take charge of their health by providing clear guidance on identifying trustworthy healthcare information and accessing reliable resources to better understand diagnoses, evaluate treatment options, and make informed decisions.
- **Increase Transparency Around Claims Denials:** Clearly explain coverage criteria in plain language—including how employer plan choices impact coverage, the role of evidence-based decisions, and the importance of providing accurate, complete information. This transparency helps members understand what's required to secure the coverage they need.
- **Ensure Digital Accessibility:** Ensure that digital health tools, telehealth platforms, and patient portals meet accessibility standards so they are usable by all members, including those with disabilities.
- **Promote Interoperability**: Champion universal compatibility between medical records, claims databases, and document systems so all providers and patients can easily share and access essential health information, regardless of software vendor.

Physical & Environmental Support

- **Support Coverage for Needs**: Address physical and environmental needs, such as specialized diets, assistive devices, and home modifications.
- **Promote Accessibility and Inclusion**: Ensure contracted facilities comply with accessibility standards and train staff on disability etiquette.

Community Inclusion & Social Drivers

- **Support Community Integration**: Offer coverage for services like accessible transportation, personal assistance, and home modifications.
- **Fund Social Engagement Programs**: Reduce isolation by supporting peer networks and accessible community activities and recreation.
- **Expand Access to Supportive Technologies:** Offer coverage for digital health tools, assistive devices—including navigation aids like AI-powered canes for individuals with vision impairments—and other innovative technologies that enhance independence, safety, and social connection.
- **Remove Financial Disincentives to Work:** Protect essential supports by phasing out benefits gradually as income rises, allowing individuals to retain critical resources while working. Ensure the phase-out process is clearly communicated and easy to understand.
- **Support Employment:** Ensure individuals with disabilities or health conditions that make employment difficult have access to job coaching, reliable transportation, and assistive technology to support meaningful employment and independence.
- **Enhance Access to Healthcare:** Partner with communities to ensure health information is available in multiple formats. Invest in outreach, transportation, language access services, and collaborative partnerships that expand access and reduce barriers for populations affected by adverse social drivers of health.

Honoring Member Voices and Choices

- **Empower Member Choice:** Streamline processes for exceptions and accommodations, and take steps to understand and respect members' unique needs and preferences.
- **Recognize Preferences:** Ensure care plans give patients the opportunity to express their care preferences and have them meaningfully reflected in coverage and treatment decisions, improving satisfaction and outcomes.
- **Maximize Flexibility:** Design benefits and policies that allow for individual choice, such as self-directed care and allowing provisions for members to decide how they spend support funds, to ensure care aligns with each member's unique needs and preferences.
- **Foster Respectful Member Experiences**: Monitor and address complaints related to disrespect, lack of autonomy, delays, wait times, and other concerns to foster a respectful and responsive environment.

Continuous Improvement

- **Expand Feedback Gathering:** In addition to traditional member surveys, seek input from families, providers, colleagues, and community stakeholders. Use informal feedback channels and advisory boards to better understand the needs of people affected by disability and adverse social drivers of health. Include frequent microsurveys to gather quick, real-time feedback and spot emerging issues.

- **Analyze Member Feedback and Implement Change:** Disaggregate member data to identify patterns and gaps in care. Use these insights to inform policy changes and guide targeted improvements that enhance access, quality, and outcomes for all members.
- **Share Denial Trends with Providers:** Develop systems that analyze and share denial trends to help providers understand why claims are being denied. Include mechanisms to disaggregate data by provider and offer this information as needed to support process improvement, reduce administrative burden, and improve access to prompt care.
- **Review Automated Tools:** Regularly audit algorithms and AI systems to ensure they do not unintentionally limit benefits or services for any group.
- **Reward Quality Outcomes:** Adopt payment models that incentivize smooth care transitions, high patient satisfaction, and measurable improvements in health outcomes.
- **Keep Your Word:** Whether you make a public commitment or a promise to an individual member, always follow through. If unforeseen circumstances such as new regulatory restrictions prevent you from doing so, be transparent about the change and clearly explain why.

NOTES

PREFACE

1. Chapman University, "Chapman Survey of American Fears 2024: Key Findings," Babbie Center for Social Research, Wilkinson College of Arts, Humanities, and Social Sciences, PDF, 2024.https://www.chapman.edu/wilkinson/research-centers/babbie-center/_files/2024-csaf-key-findings-final.pdf
2. Lad SP, Santarelli JG, Patil CG, Steinberg GK, Boakye M. National trends in spinal arteriovenous malformations. Neurosurg Focus. 2009 Jan;26(1):1-5. doi: 10.3171/FOC.2009.26.1.E10. PMID: 19228104 https://thejns.org/focus/view/journals/neurosurg-focus/26/1/article-p1.pdf.

INTRODUCTION

1. Adelina Comas-Herrera, Pedro Gozalo, Andrew W. Dick, and Joan Costa-Font, "The Impact of Ownership Type on COVID-19 Mortality in English and U.S. Nursing Homes: Evidence from a New Survey," *International Journal for Quality in Health Care* 36, no. 3 (2024): mzae078, https://doi.org/10.1093/intqhc/mzae078.
2. Angela Coulter and John Oldham, "Person-Centred Care: What Is It and How Do We Get There?" *Future Hospital Journal* 3, no. 2 (2016): 114–116, https://pmc.ncbi.nlm.nih.gov/articles/PMC6465833/.
3. Gianpaolo Tomaselli et al., "Person-Centered Care from a Relational Ethics Perspective for the Chronically Ill," Frontiers in Public Health 8, no. 5 (2020), https://www.frontiersin.org/journals/public-health/articles/10.3389/fpubh.2020.00044/full.
4. Tomaselli et al.; Alessandra Giusti et al., 'The Empirical Evidence Underpinning the Concept and Practice of Person-Centred Care for Serious Illness: A Systematic Review," BMJ Global Health 5, no. 12 (2020), https://gh.bmj.com/content/5/12/e003330.
5. Coulter and Oldham, 114–116; Anam Ahmed, "Person-Centred Care in Primary Care: What Works for Whom, How and in What Circumstances?" *Health and Social Care in the Community* 30, no. 6 (2022), https://onlinelibrary.wiley.com/doi/10.1111/hsc.13913.
6. https://picker.org/who-we-are/the-picker-principles-of-person-centred-care/.
7. https://declarationforindependence.org/about-us/.

1. FROM PARTY MODE TO PATIENT

1. Michael Anne Kyle and Austin B. Frakt, "Patient Administrative Burden in the US Health Care System," *Health Services Research* 56, no. 5 (October 2021): 755–65, https://pubmed.ncbi.nlm.nih.gov/34498259/.
2. Nomi S. Weiss-Laxer etal., "Families as a Cornerstone in 21st Century Public Health: Recommendations for Research, Education, Policy, and Practice," *Frontiers in Public Health* 8 (2020): article 503, https://doi.org/10.3389/fpubh.2020.00503.
3. SimaMarzbanetal., "Impact of Patient Engagement on Healthcare Quality: A Scoping Review," *Journal of Patient Experience* 9 (September 2022): article 23743735221125439, https://doi.org/10.1177/23743735221125439.
4. Myriam Deveugele, "Communication Training: Skills and Beyond," *Patient Education and Counseling* 98, no. 10 (October 2015): 1287–91, https://doi.org/10.1016/j.pec.2015.08.011. (PubMed PMID: 26298220.)
5. HealthCentral, "What You Told Us About Medical Gaslighting," *HealthCentral*, August 25, 2023, updated September 28, 2023, https://www.healthcentral.com/chronic-health/what-you-told-us-about-medical-gaslighting.
6. Allyson C. Bontempo, John M. Bontempo, and Paul R. Duberstein, "Ignored, Dismissed, and Minimized: Understanding the Harmful Consequences of Invalidation in Health Care—A Systematic Meta-Synthesis of Qualitative Research," *Psychological Bulletin* 151, no. 4 (April 2025): 399–427, https://pubmed.ncbi.nlm.nih.gov/40310228
7. The Joint Commission, *"Patient Safety Topics,"* The Joint Commission, https://www.jointcommission.org/resources/patient-safety-topics/.
8. CARF International, *"Resources for the Public,"* CARF International, https://carf.org/resources/public/
9. Model Systems Knowledge Translation Center, *"Model Systems Knowledge Translation Center,"* https://msktc.org/.
10. U.S. National Library of Medicine, *"Health Topics,"* MedlinePlus, https://medlineplus.gov/healthtopics.html.
11. National Institutes of Health, *"Health Information,"* National Institutes of Health, https://www.nih.gov/health-information.

2. FINDING MY DREAM DOCTOR

1. ArielaM.Freedman, KathleenR.Miner, KatharinaV.Echt, and RuthParker, "Amplifying Diffusion of Health Information in Low-Literate Populations through Adult Education Health Literacy Classes," *Journal of Health Communication*, supplement 3 (2011): 119–33, https://doi.org/10.1080/10810730.2011.604706.
2. Sima Babaei and Shahla Abolhasani, "Family's Supportive Behaviors in the Care of the Patient Admitted to the Cardiac Care Unit: A Qualitative Study,"

Journal of Caring Sciences 9, no. 2 (June 2020): 80–86, https://doi.org/10.34172/jcs.2020.012.

3. Kaiser Family Foundation, "Claims Denials and Appeals in ACA Marketplace Plans in 2023," *KFF*, January2025, https://www.kff.org/private-insurance/issue-brief/claims-denials-and-appeals-in-aca-marketplace-plans-in-2023/

4. Premier Inc., "Claims Adjudication Costs Providers $25.7Billion–$18Billion Is Potentially Unnecessary Expense," *Premier Newsroom*, February24,2025, https://premierinc.com/newsroom/policy/claims-adjudication-costs-providers-257-billion-18-billion-is-potentially-unnecessary-expense

5. Kaiser Family Foundation, *Claims Denials and Appeals*, 2025.

6. Saendy Jung and Rachel H. McDowell, "Abandonment," in *StatPearls* (Treasure Island, FL: StatPearls Publishing, January 2025), https://www.ncbi.nlm.nih.gov/books/NBK563285/.

7. Lauren Parr, "45 Statistics on Patient Reviews for Healthcare Professionals," RepuGen, April 30, 2024, https://www.repugen.com/blog/statistics-on-patient-reviews-for-healthcare-professionals.

8. Zejia A. Yu and Michelle B. Gorgone, " Pay-for-Performance and Value-Based Care," StatPearls, May 2, 2024, https://www.ncbi.nlm.nih.gov/books/NBK607995/.

9. Linda Ljungholm et al., "What Is Needed for Continuity of Care and How Can We Achieve It? Perceptions Among Multiprofessionals on the Chronic Care Trajectory," *BMC Health Services Research* 22, no. 1: 686, https://pmc.ncbi.nlm.nih.gov/articles/PMC9125858/.

10. Janet C. Long etal., "Needs of People with Rare Diseases That Can Be Supported by Electronic Resources: A Scoping Review," *BMJ Open* 12, no. 9 (2022): e060394, https://doi.org/10.1136/bmjopen-2021-060394.

3. SURGERY AND THE CITY

1. MichaelA.Rosen, DeborahDiazGranados, AaronS.Dietz, LaurenE.Benishek, DavidThompson, PeterJ.Pronovost, and SallieJ.Weaver, "Teamwork in Healthcare: Key Discoveries Enabling Safer, High-Quality Care," *American Psychologist* 73, no. 4 (May–June2018): 433–50, https://doi.org/10.1037/amp0000298.

2. Sarah Morey and Alison Steven, "The Transition to 'Patienthood,' the Contribution of the Nursing Assistant: A Grounded Theory Study," *Journal of Patient Experience* 7, no. 6: 1693–1700, https://pmc.ncbi.nlm.nih.gov/articles/PMC7786661/.

3. Hogikyan ND, Kana LA, Shuman AG, Firn JI. Patient perceptions of trust formation in the surgeon-patient relationship: A thematic analysis. Patient Educ Couns. 2021 Sep;104(9):2338-2343. doi: 10.1016/j.pec.2021.02.002. Epub 2021 Feb 5. PMID: 33583655; PMCID: PMC12044868.

4. Al Nou'mani J, Al Alawi AM, Al-Maqbali JS, Al Abri N, Al Sabbri M. Prevalence, Recognition, and Risk Factors of Constipation among Medically Hospi-

talized Patients: A Cohort Prospective Study. Medicina (Kaunas). 2023 Jul 23;59(7):1347. doi: 10.3390/medicina59071347. PMID: 37512158; PMCID: PMC10385149.

5. Jawahar Al Nou'mani etal., "Prevalence, Recognition, and Risk Factors of Constipation among Medically Hospitalized Patients: A Cohort Prospective Study," *Medicina* 59, no.7 (2023): article1347, https://doi.org/10.3390/medicina59071347.

6. Mandy Fader etal., "Technology for Managing Incontinence: What Are the Research Priorities?," *Proceedings of the Institution of Mechanical Engineers, Part H: Journal of Engineering in Medicine* 238, no. 6 (June 2024): 688–703, https://doi.org/10.1177/09544119241233639.

7. Fahmida Hossain, Ezra Gabbay, and Joseph J. Fins, "Clinical Ethics and the Observant Jewish and Muslim Patient: Shared Theocentric Perspectives in Practice," *Cambridge Quarterly of Healthcare Ethics* 34, no. 2 (April 2025): 247–63, https://doi.org/10.1017/S0963180124000379.

4. INPATIENT REHAB

1. Hoffmann T, Bakhit M, Michaleff Z. Shared decision making and physical therapy: What, when, how, and why? Braz J Phys Ther. 2022 Jan-Feb;26(1):100382. doi: 10.1016/j.bjpt.2021.100382. Epub 2022 Jan 1, https://pubmed.ncbi.nlm.nih.gov/35063699/.

2. Dossa A, Bokhour B, Hoenig H. Care transitions from the hospital to home for patients with mobility impairments: patient and family caregiver experiences. Rehabil Nurs. 2012 Nov-Dec;37(6):277-85. doi: 10.1002/rnj.047. Epub 2012 Jun 29. PMID: 23212952 https://pubmed.ncbi.nlm.nih.gov/23212952/.

3. DorothyE.Stubbe, "Practicing Cultural Competence and Cultural Humility in the Care of Diverse Patients," *Focus* 18, no.1 (January 2020): 49–51, https://doi.org/10.1176/appi.focus.20190041.

4. LindaLjungholm, AnetteEdin-Liljegren, MirjamEkstedt, and CharlotteKlinga, "What Is Needed for Continuity of Care and How Can We Achieve It? – Perceptions among Multiprofessionals on the Chronic Care Trajectory," *BMC Health Services Research* 22, article686 (2022), https://doi.org/10.1186/s12913-022-08023-0.

5. Sasha Shepperd, Natasha A. Lannin, Lindy M. Clemson, Annie McCluskey, Ian D. Cameron, and Sarah L. Barras, "Discharge Planning from Hospital to Home," *Cochrane Database of Systematic Reviews*, no. 1 (January 31, 2013): CD000313, https://doi.org/10.1002/14651858.CD000313.pub4.

6. NaifAlzahrani, "The Effect of Hospitalization on Patients' Emotional and Psychological Well-Being among Adult Patients: An Integrative Review," *Applied Nursing Research* 61 (October 2021): 151488, https://doi.org/10.1016/j.apnr.2021.151488.

7. The Joint Commission, *Advancing Effective Communication, Cultural Competence, and Patient- and Family-Centered Care: A Roadmap for Hospitals* (Oakbrook Terrace, IL: The Joint Commission, 2022), https://www.jointcommission.org/-/media/tjc/documents/resources/patient-safety-topics/health-equity/aroadmapforhospitalsfinalversion727pdf.pdf.

5. NEW BODY, "WHO DIS?"

1. Tyler N, Hodkinson A, Planner C, et al. Transitional Care Interventions From Hospital to Community to Reduce Health Care Use and Improve Patient Outcomes: A Systematic Review and Network Meta-Analysis. JAMA Netw Open. 2023;6(11):e2344825. doi:10.1001/jamanetworkopen.2023.44825 https://pubmed.ncbi.nlm.nih.gov/38032642/.
2. StephanieA.Bird, "Assessing Accessibility: An Investigation into Variations in ADA Compliance Across the US," *Araneum: Richmond Journal of American & Global Affairs* 2, no. 2 (2025): article4, https://doi.org/10.26736/ar.02.02.01.
3. Ledford CJW, Cafferty LA, Lee E, Hayes HC, Ede DC, Hodges BP, Whitebloom GC, Walsh DW, Wilkins T. How Social Connectedness Helps Patients Stay Home After Hospital at Home Enrollment: A Mixed Methods Study. J Gen Intern Med. 2024 Nov;39(14):2671-2678. doi: 10.1007/s11606-024-08785-9. Epub 2024 May 9. PMID: 38724740; PMCID: PMC11534937 https://pubmed.ncbi.nlm.nih.gov/38724740/.
4. Anjali J. Forber-Pratt, Gabriel J. Merrin, Carlyn O. Mueller, Larry R. Price, and Heather Hensman Kettrey, "Initial Factor Exploration of Disability Identity," *Rehabilitation Psychology* 65, no.1 (February 2020): 1–10, https://doi.org/10.1037/rep0000308.

6. HELP DESK CENTRAL

1. U.S. Bureau of Labor Statistics, *Persons with a Disability: Labor Force Characteristics — 2023*, news release, June 26, 2024, https://www.bls.gov/news.release/pdf/disabl.pdf.
2. Choi, G., Seo, J. Accessibility, Usability, and Universal Design for Learning: Discussion of Three Key LX/UX Elements for Inclusive Learning Design. *TechTrends* 68, 936–945 (2024). https://doi.org/10.1007/s11528-024-00987-6.
3. Borges CM, Pollock JC, Crowley M, Purandare R, Sparano J, Spike K. Social capital or vulnerability: Which has the stronger connection with selected U.S. health outcomes? SSM Popul Health. 2021 May 5;15:100812. doi: 10.1016/j.ssmph.2021.100812. PMID: 34141850; PMCID: PMC8188049.
4. Tyler N, Hodkinson A, Planner C, Angelakis I, Keyworth C, Hall A, Jones PP, Wright OG, Keers R, Blakeman T, Panagioti M. Transitional Care Interventions From Hospital to Community to Reduce Health Care Use and Improve Patient Outcomes: A Systematic Review and Network Meta-Analysis. JAMA Netw

Open. 2023 Nov 1;6(11):e2344825. doi: 10.1001/jamanet-workopen.2023.44825. PMID: 38032642; PMCID: PMC10690480.

5. Helena Hansen, Philippe Bourgois, and Ernest Drucker, "Pathologizing Poverty: New Forms of Diagnosis, Disability, and Structural Stigma under Welfare Reform," *Social Science & Medicine* 103 (2014): 76–83, https://doi.org/10.1016/j.socscimed.2013.06.033.

7. FINDING YOUR SWEET SPOT

1. Elizabeth Zimmermann, "Mayo Clinic Researchers Demonstrate Value of Second Opinions," Mayo Clinic, April 4, 2017, https://newsnetwork.mayoclinic.org/discussion/mayo-clinic-researchers-demonstrate-value-of-second-opinions/.

2. S.Bowman, "Impact of Electronic Health Record Systems on Information Integrity: Quality and Safety Implications," *Perspectives in Health Information Management* 10 (Fall 2013): 1c, https://www.ncbi.nlm.nih.gov/pmc/articles/PMC3797550.

3. Eunjung Lim, Jill Miyamura, and JohnJ.Chen, "Racial/Ethnic-Specific Reference Intervals for Common Laboratory Tests: A Comparison among Asians, Blacks, Hispanics, and White," *Hawaii Journal of Medicine & Public Health* 74, no.9 (September2015): 302–10, https://www.ncbi.nlm.nih.gov/pmc/articles/PMC4578165.

4. Christophers, L., Torok, Z., Trayer, A. *et al.* Interdisciplinary teamworking in rehabilitation: experiences of change initiators in a national rehabilitation hospital. *BMC Health Serv Res* 25, 651 (2025). https://doi.org/10.1186/s12913-025-12795-6.

5. Rohwer, A., Toews, I., Uwimana-Nicol, J. *et al.* Models of integrated care for multi-morbidity assessed in systematic reviews: a scoping review. *BMC Health Serv Res* 23, 894 (2023). https://doi.org/10.1186/s12913-023-09894-7.

6. Diagnostic Errors, *PSNet* [Internet], Rockville, MD: Agency for Healthcare Research and Quality, U.S. Department of Health and Human Services, 2019, https://psnet.ahrq.gov/primer/diagnostic-errors.

7. Mohamad Aljofan etal., "The Rate of Medication Nonadherence and Influencing Factors: A Systematic Review," *Electronic Journal of General Medicine* 20, no.3 (May 1, 2023): em471, https://doi.org/10.29333/ejgm/12946.

8. I'M STILL STANDING

1. JongSeokAhn, SangwonShin, Su-AYang, EunKyungPark, KiHwanKim, SooIckCho, Chan-YoungOck, and SeokhwiKim, "Artificial Intelligence in Breast Cancer Diagnosis and Personalized Medicine," *Journal of Breast Cancer* 26, no.5 (October2023): 405–35, https://www.ncbi.nlm.nih.gov/pmc/articles/PMC10625863.

2. Michael D. Abramoff, Tinglong Dai, and James Zou, "Scaling Adoption of Medical AI — Reimbursement from Value-Based Care and Fee-for-Service Perspectives," *AI in Precision Cardiovascular Medicine*, published April 12, 2024, https://doi.org/10.1056/AIpc2400083.

3. Chustecki M, Benefits and Risks of AI in Health Care: Narrative Review, Interact J Med Res 2024;13:e53616, https://www.i-jmr.org/2024/1/e53616, DOI: 10.2196/53616.

4. MoritzReis, FlorianReis, and WilfriedKunde, "Public Perception of Physicians Who Use Artificial Intelligence," *JAMA Network Open* 8, no.7 (July 1, 2025): e2521643, https://doi.org/10.1001/jamanetworkopen.2025.21643. (PubMed PMID:40674054; PMCID:PMC12272287).

9. SHOW ME THE MONEY

1. *Peterson-KFF Health System Tracker*, "How Has U.S. Spending on Healthcare Changed Over Time?" chart collection (Peterson Center on Healthcare and KFF, 2024), https://www.healthsystemtracker.org/chart-collection/u-s-spending-healthcare-changed-time/.

2. DavidBlumenthal, EvanD.Gumas, ArnavShah, MuniraZ.Gunja, and ReginaldD.WilliamsII, *Mirror, Mirror2024: A Portrait of the Failing U.S. Health System* (New York: The Commonwealth Fund, September19,2024), https://www.commonwealthfund.org/publications/fund-reports/2024/sep/mirror-mirror-2024.

3. Eric C. Schneider, Arnav Shah, Melinda Abrams, and Laurie Zephyrin, *Mirror, Mirror 2024: Reflecting Poorly—Health Care in the U.S. Compared to Other High-Income Countries* (New York: The Commonwealth Fund, September 2024), https://www.commonwealthfund.org/publications/fund-reports/2024/sep/mirror-mirror-2024.

4. National Association of Insurance Commissioners, *2024 Annual Health Industry Commentary* (Kansas City, MO: NAIC, 2024), https://content.naic.org/sites/default/files/2024-annual-health-industry-commentary.pdf.

5. AHIP (America's Health Insurance Plans), "Where Does Your Health Care Dollar Go?," *AHIP*, October 24, 2024, https://www.ahip.org/resources/where-does-your-health-care-dollar-go.

6. Kaiser Family Foundation, *"What to Know About Medicare Spending and Financing,"* KFF, November2022, https://www.kff.org/medicare/issue-brief/what-to-know-about-medicare-spending-and-financing/.

7. NikhilR. Sahni, BrookeIstvan, HeatherBello Thornhill, KarenE. Joynt-Maddox, DavidCutler, and EzekielJ.Emanuel, "Availability of Consistent, Reliable, and Actionable Public Data on US Hospital Administrative Expenses," *Health Affairs Scholar* 3, no.5 (May22,2025): qxaf069, https://www.ncbi.nlm.nih.gov/pmc/articles/PMC12096959.

8. KarenEggleston, Yu-ChuShen, JosephLau, ChristopherH.Schmid, and JiaChan, "Hospital Ownership and Quality of Care: What Explains the Different Results in the Literature?," *Health Economics* 17, no.12 (December2008): 1345–62, https://pubmed.ncbi.nlm.nih.gov/18186547.

9. RAND Corporation, "Prescription Drug Prices in the U.S. Are 2.78 Times Those in Other Countries," *RAND News Release*, February 1, 2024, https://www.rand.org/news/press/2024/02/01.html.

10. Web Golinkin, "Why Does an $84,000 Drug in the U.S. Cost Less Than $1,000 in India," *Forbes*, October23,2024, https://www.forbes.com/sites/forbesbooksauthors/2024/10/23/why-does-an-84000-drug-in-the-us-cost-less-than-1000-in-india/.

11. Grace Sparks, AshleyKirzinger, AlexMontero, IsabelleValdes, and LizHamel, "Public Opinion on Prescription Drugs and Their Prices," *KFF*, October4,2024, https://www.kff.org/health-costs/poll-finding/public-opinion-on-prescription-drugs-and-their-prices/.

12. BenjaminN. Rome etal., "Trends in Prescription Drug Launch Prices, 2008–2021," *JAMA* 327, no. 22 (June 7, 2022): 2203–05, https://doi.org/10.1001/jama.2022.6180.

13. Reuters, "Prices for new U.S. drugs doubled in 4 years as focus on rare disease grows," *Reuters*, May 22, 2025, https://www.reuters.com/business/healthcare-pharmaceuticals/prices-new-us-drugs-doubled-4-years-focus-rare-disease-grows-2025-05-22/.

14. AHIP (America's Health Insurance Plans), *Prior Authorization: Reforming a Broken System* (Washington, DC: AHIP, June2025), https://ahiporg-production.s3.amazonaws.com/documents/202506_AHIP_Report_Prior_Authorization-final.pdf.

MOVING FORWARD

1. Maria J. Santana, Kimberly Manalili, RachelJ.Jolley, Sandra Zelinsky, Hude Quan, and Mingshan Lu, "How to Practice Person-Centred Care: A Conceptual Framework," *Health Expectations* 21, no.2 (April 2018): 429–40, https://doi.org/10.1111/hex.12640.

THANK YOU
FOR READING MY BOOK!

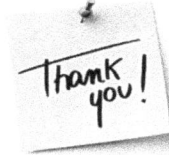

ACCESS ADDITIONAL RESOURCES

Thank you for investing your time in this book. This isn't the end of the conversation—it's just the beginning. I've gathered a few resources to help you continue exploring person-centered care.

Scan the QR Code:

Before you go, if this book gave you a chuckle, a new outlook, or even a fun break from reading medical records, please consider leaving your invaluable review on Amazon.com or another site. Your feedback helps other readers discover these stories and inspires me to keep writing. Thank you!

www.ingramcontent.com/pod-product-compliance
Lightning Source LLC
Chambersburg PA
CBHW050647270326
41927CB00012B/2917